Buy Basal
Thermometer
(eg. one does not
work on this)

Homework Chap. 4   *40-54
Meeting Chap. 10   *203
#2   p. 88 chart

for
meeting { Chap. 6
#3
          #4 April 10

The Art of
Natural Family Planning

Mr. + Mrs. Raymond Massé

Practical Applications Workbook $2.00

For self-instruction at home, readers will find this workbook of 20 charts plus answers sheet invaluable. For use with this manual and thus sold only to manual owners. Please clip this coupon and send with check. Users have said this workbook is really helpful.

Dear CCL: Here's our membership contribution to help make NFP information more available. Please send us the *CCL News* (6 times a year) so we can keep up to date on any new developments in natural family planning.

Enclosed is our check for $10.00 for a year's membership.

Please make checks payable to Couple to Couple League. Contributions to CCL are tax deductible. Please print name and address as you want the *CCL News* addressed to you.

Name_____ Date _____

Street _____

City _____ State _____ Zip Code _____

Other Materials: Basal temperature thermometers, daily observation charts and other books related to parenting can also be purchased from the CCL national office. Please write for complete materials list.

This page is for use by couples who are learning NFP by self-instruction rather than through attendance at CCL classes.

The Art of
Natural Family Planning

by
John and Sheila Kippley

Foreward by Konald A. Prem, M.D.

Published by:

The Couple to Couple League
International Inc.

P.O. Box 11084
Cincinnati, OH 45211

Addresses of other organizations referred to in the text:

La Leche League International (LLLI)
9616 Minneapolis Avenue
Franklin Park, Ill. 60131
Counseling telephone number at any time: (312) 455-7730

ICEA Supplies Center
1414 N.W. 85th Street
Seattle, Wash. 98117

Drawings on page 30, 32 and 39 by Anita Hassel

All net proceeds from the sale of this book go to the Couple to Couple League International, Inc., a non-profit organization to assist couples with the successful practice of natural family planning.

First Edition, Revised; Fifth Printing

Cataloging Data   ISBN 0-9601036-2-7

Kippley, John F. and Sheila K.
The Art of Natural Family Planning.
Includes bibliography.

1. Natural Family Planning.   2. Birth Control.
3. Sexual Morality.   4. Breast-feeding.

Acknowledgments

First and foremost, a special note of thanks must be given to Konald A. Prem, M.D. Without his expertise and experience this manual would not be the same and might not exist at all. Dr. Prem was one of the few who kept the light of natural family planning switched on when most of his medical colleagues had opted for the contraceptive approach. He helped us in starting the Couple to Couple League, has given unstintingly of his time to the Twin Cities CCL chapter, and has provided us with what seems to be most of what we have learned about natural family planning. Furthermore, he reviewed the biologically oriented chapters of this book in great detail and suggested numerous alterations to make it both more accurate and more readable.

Secondly, we want to express our indebtedness to the pioneers whose work made this manual possible—to Mary Putnam Jacobi, a women's rights physician who in 1876 was the first to provide an exact description of basal temperature changes during the menstrual cycle; to Wilhelm Hillebrand, a German Catholic priest who was the first to use basal temperature changes to determine the infertile period; to Drs. Kyusaku Ogino and Hermann Knaus for their discoveries about ovulation in the 1920s; to Dr. Edward F. Keefe for his publications about the cervix as an indicator of fertility; to Dr. John Marshall of England for his writings on temperature theory; to Drs. Evelyn and John Billings for their work in developing rules of thumb to make the observation of cervical mucus more useful as an indicator of fertility; to Dr. Claude Lanctot, who early recognized and promoted the value of having trained couples instruct others about natural family planning; to the pioneer organizations of couples who have helped so many others during the last decade; to La Leche League for its educational work about the benefits of breast-feeding.

Thirdly, we want to acknowledge the help we have received from those who reviewed our preliminary edition and sent us their comments

v

and suggestions: Dr. Paul Busam, Rev. Marc Calegari, S.J., Roger and Peggy Carter, Bill and Joan Cossette, Rose Gioiosa, Barbara Gross, Gretchen Healy, Dr. Tom Hilgers, Terry and Nancy Hornback, Dr. Claude and Anne Lanctot, Dr. John McCarthy, Fr. John Mucharski, Dr. Tom Nabors, Rev. Stephen Schneider, O.F.M., Frank and Connie Sheehan, Dr. Pierre Slightam, Paul and Carol Vitek, and Pat Yearian. Their suggestions have made the task of writing this manual much easier, but the final responsibility for the present book must remain with us.

We also acknowledge the kind permission to quote from the following copyrighted sources: Max Levin, "Sexual Fulfillment with Rhythm," *Marriage,* June 1966; Dr. Paul Marx, O.S.B., *The Death Peddlers: War on the Unborn,* Collegeville, Minn.: St. John's University Press, 1971; and Michael F. Valente, *Sex: The Radical View of a Catholic Theologian,* New York: The Bruce Publishing Company, 1970.

Finally, we thank all those couples who have indicated in one way or another their satisfaction with and successful use of the preliminary edition of this book. Such comments have been helpful indeed in providing the stimulus to complete the present edition in the hopes of making adequate information about natural family planning available to all who desire it.

John and Sheila Kippley
The Couple to Couple League
P.O. Box 11084
Cincinnati, Ohio 45211
Phone: (513) 661-7612

Contents

Foreword

Natural family planning has come of age. It is therefore with great pleasure that I introduce this book to its readers.

Throughout the history of man, a natural but limited form of child spacing has been available through long term breast-feeding. However, the introduction of bottle feeding with cow's milk and milk substitutes deprived mothers of the natural infertility derived from successful long term lactation. Today only two groups of women still enjoy that period of prolonged postpartum relative infertility: 1) those in cultures in which the practice of nursing described in this book as "ecological breast-feeding" continues and 2) those who have learned this practice despite the lack of cultural support. Since it is scientifically established that maternal breast milk is the best infant food and that the breast-feeding pattern described in this manual definitely provides an extended period of infertility, it is of distinct value that this form of breast-feeding is described and recommended to those interested in natural family planning. On the average, such a nursing pattern may provide 18 to 30 months spacing between births without supplemental spacing methods.

However, most couples today seek to regulate conception beyond the possibilities offered by breast-feeding and many are interested in natural methods. The first real help for those interested in natural family planning became available in the 1930's through the independent research of Doctors Kyusaku Ogino in Japan and Hermann Knaus in Austria. These pioneers in reproductive physiology discovered that ovulation occurs approximately two weeks prior to the following menstruation. From their observations they formulated certain rules of thumb for periodic coital abstinence that became known as "rhythm." Because their systems did not sufficiently consider the various forms of menstrual irregularity experienced by many women, many couples were disillusioned by repeated failures. Although the reasons for these failures are now better understood, rhythm is no longer recommended by natural family planners. It is still recognized, however, for what it was: the first natural family planning system in the history of mankind based upon scientific study and oriented toward an educated awareness of fertility.

The efficiency of natural family planning systems was aided immensely by the discovery that the hormone progesterone, produced by the ovary after ovulation, caused an easily measured elevation of the basal body temperature which persisted until menstruation. Observations of signs and symptoms of ovulation such as ovulation pain (Mittelschmerz), pelvic pressure, changes in the amount and physical characteristics of cervical mucus and changes in cervical os dilatation led to the development of the sympto-thermal method of natural family planning. During the 1950's and 1960's, while studying the reasons for rhythm failures by application of the basal body temperatures graph, I assisted many couples to develop a high degree of proficiency using the sympto-thermal methods for family limitation. Published studies referred to in this manual have shown that a sophisticated practice of the sympto-thermal method can achieve a use-effectiveness rate comparable to or better than most artificial contraceptive methods except sterilization and the original high dose combined oral contraceptive pills.

Although there is no scientific justification for negative comments about the effectiveness of the sympto-thermal method of natural family planning, it is obvious that its effectiveness for any given couple will depend upon several factors: the couple must learn it, understand it, and above all be motivated to make it work. Many couples so motivated have asked in the past and are asking with increasing frequency today this question: "Where can we learn about natural family planning?"

In 1962 the late Doctor Carl Hartman, an eminent reproductive physiologist, wrote in his compendium of human reproduction, *Science and the Safe Period*—"no physician should refuse to teach the best methods of calculating the fertile period to patients requesting the instruction." Unfortunately, the majority of my medical colleagues have ignored this advice: only a few have remained informed and are knowledgeable about the scientific developments in natural family planning. Because of their apathy and lack of information, some physicians attempt to persuade patients to abandon natural family planning in favor of sterilization or the artificial methods.

This widespread physician apathy toward natural family planning provided the stimulus to interested married couples and physicians to organize teaching teams to instruct other interested couples outside the traditional medical setting. A few such groups began to function in the 1960's in certain areas of the country. In 1971 John and Sheila Kippley approached me and with my cooperation established the Couple to Couple League, a volunteer organization to provide the effective teaching of natural family planning on a nationwide basis. In addition, they saw the need for an authoritative instruction manual. I was pleased to cooperate in both of these projects and allowed them to use many of the informative fertility graphs I had collected over more than 20 years of interest and experience in the sympto-thermal method.

The normal instructional format for the interested couple combines formal classes such as those taught by the Couple to Couple League and the personal study of an authoritative manual. However, such an opportunity is not available to all today. While a book is no substitute for adequate personalized instruction, this manual can be used for self-instruction in geographic areas where formal classes are not yet available. Serving as a reliable source of information for married couples and physicians alike, it is an indispensable aid to the successful practice of the art of natural family planning.

Konald A. Prem, M.D.
Professor
Department of Obstetrics & Gynecology
University of Minnesota

Introduction

The title of this manual, *The Art of Natural Family Planning,* was chosen very deliberately. In practice, natural family planning is an art. It involves a certain amount of skill in observing and interpreting the monthly signs. It is relatively simple, but still it has to be learned. It involves the use of reason in the learning process and in making practical judgments. It involves the use of freedom in making decisions about whether to express mutual marital affection in the coital embrace or in some other way.

As in any art, one's practice of natural family planning improves through experience. It doesn't require any genius to become skilled in this art, but it does require a little practice in the observation and interpretation of signs in order for the couple to feel really comfortable with it. In a way it is like swimming. The person who says "I can't swim and I can't learn and therefore I won't try" will never develop the art of swimming with those attitudes. The person who has an open attitude, follows directions, and practices soon feels comfortable swimming: An art has been learned. So also with natural family planning.

Purpose

The primary purpose of this manual is to help people to develop the art of natural family planning. It can also be used by those, such as doctors, who simply want more information, but it is designed especially for typical couples with common, ordinary concerns about family planning. This manual is intended to help those couples in two ways.

First of all, the manual is as complete a handbook on the various methods of natural family planning as the average couple can buy or can understand. Presumably, medical textbooks are more complete, but they are too expensive and too detailed for most people. This manual was written because the authors formerly had to refer interested couples to several different books and publications for information about various aspects of natural family planning. There wasn't any single book that had everything in it that we felt was essential for a comprehensive package of natural family planning. Thus, this manual is more complete than anything we knew of when we wrote it.

Secondly, the manual is more than a convenient handbook on the biological aspects of natural family planning. It was not our intention simply to produce a book about the anatomy and physiology of the female reproduction system. We felt that it was necessary to spend some time examining attitudes toward natural family planning. The day is fortunately past when scientists were supposed to inform others about fact after fact without ever making any moral evaluations; and if there is any area of human concern where the use of scientific facts is closely related to morality, it is in sexual behavior and the transmission of life. The reader should thus realize that every book about sex or birth control expresses the convictions of its author, even if that conviction is that sex is without moral consequence. It is our experience that some writers on this subject cloak their values and their real reasons for writing; we have decided on a policy of openness, even if that means that some readers will reject us.

Our comments about attitudes and morality are intended first of all to help the people who share our convictions. Frequently, such people feel rather lonely today, and they are looking for a way to express their own convictions. Secondly, these comments are intended to raise some questions for others who are open to serious thought about these matters. In our present society, it is difficult to hear these questions raised, and we are convinced that many couples will come to agree with us after further reflection on the values involved. Lastly, a discussion of attitudes is important because in a great many human efforts the key to success is attitude. When the coach of a winning team is asked for the reasons, he almost always names a "can do" attitude as one of his most important ingredients. In this manual, we have assembled accurate information about the scientific facts and explained the attitudes that make for success. We think that with this combination every couple can have a winning effort.

However, the manual is not intended to encourage people to stop having babies. Even though the methods of natural family planning are themselves in accord with the order of God's creation, they can be used selfishly. The advertising industry has subtly developed rather expensive tastes in many of us, and it can be a real temptation to postpone pregnancy or limit our family size more in the interests of materialism than anything else.

At the same time, it is recognized that many couples have what they think are sufficiently serious reasons for wanting to space out or to avoid another pregnancy. Such couples will find in this manual the ways of family planning that are in accord with God's design for human sexuality.

Fertility Awareness

The form of natural family planning that is described in this manual is essentially a system of observing, recording, and interpreting facts about what is happening within a woman's body during her monthly cycle. As such, the information can be used by couples who *want* a baby and by others who desire to *avoid* pregnancy. Those whose natural family planning takes the form of complete abstinence from sexual intercourse rather obviously do not need this information for family planning purposes. However, we know of a group of women in a religious order who became skilled in making some of these observations for the purpose of greater self-knowledge. They found it quite helpful to be able to relate changes of mood to the phases within their menstrual cycles. The same would certainly hold true for married women as well.

Every woman has a periodic cycle, usually about a month long, during which she becomes fertile* and then becomes naturally infertile*. There are certain bodily signs that occur just before, during, and after the fertile phase of her cycle. The couple using natural family planning observe and interpret these signs to know when the wife is fertile and when she is infertile. If they want a pregnancy, they have sexual intercourse at the most fertile time; and if they wish to avoid pregnancy, they avoid genital contact during the fertile phase. As we shall explain more fully in later chapters, this does not mean that they shun all show of affection, but it does exclude contact of the sexual organs.

Another aspect of natural family planning is the relationship between ecological breast-feeding and an extended period of natural infertility (the term "ecological breast-feeding" is fully explained in Chapter 7). This manual differs from most books on family planning because it goes into some detail about the proper kind of breast-feeding that provides this form of natural infertility. It also describes various cultural practices that can upset this ecological relationship between mother and baby.

The art of natural family planning that is described and recommended in this manual differs significantly from the system that was known for years as the "calendar rhythm method" or simply "rhythm." The older calendar rhythm made insufficient allowances for irregularity in the woman's monthly cycle and the woman's own individual ovulation pattern. As a method it had a failure rate that was high enough to be

* For the meaning of words, see the Glossary of Terms.

very discouraging to a good number of married couples. The old rhythm system was based on the research reported by Dr. Kyusaku Ogino (1930, Japan) and Dr. Hermann Knaus (1929, Austria), who discovered that a woman ovulates (becomes fertile) about two weeks before the beginning of her next menstrual period. In the forty-odd years since then, much additional information has been discovered about the changes that take place in a woman's body during the fertile part of her monthly cycle. No one seriously involved in natural family planning today recommends the use of the Ogino-Knaus rhythm, and the criticisms of it should not be made about the methods described in this manual. At the same time, it should be recognized that the Ogino-Knaus rhythm could be effective for about 80 percent of married couples if they were willing to abide by its rules; properly used, it could be about as effective as the mechanical contraceptives available during the years before the Pill.

The Couple to Couple League

The Couple to Couple League is a nondenominational, nonprofit organization dedicated to helping couples develop the art of natural family planning. It began in the fall of 1971 when the authors of this manual secured the assistance of Dr. Konald Prem and began offering what they hoped would be a regularly recurring series of four meetings on natural family planning. At the prescribed time for the beginning of the first meeting in a school library in Shoreview, a suburb north of St. Paul, Minnesota, exactly one person, a lone man, was in attendance. The decision to start promptly at eight o'clock was reconsidered on queasy stomachs,—and within ten minutes or so about thirty people filled the room. Thus, the League was born. Succeeding meetings have started on time, and we think we have seen an ever increasing interest in the CCL approach to teaching natural family planning.

The CCL Manual

This manual came into being not as part of a master plan but rather out of the necessity of circumstances. For one thing, we were concerned that we had to recommend about five different books as supplementary reading, each of them covering one aspect of the system we were teaching. However, the more immediate circumstance was that we knew we would be leaving the St. Paul area in a few months. When we asked some other couples to carry on the work of CCL, we promised them lesson plans for the meetings plus this manual. The original mimeographed printing was only 100 copies, for it was our intention to send these copies to people with much experience in the field of natural family planning for their comments and then to produce immediately a revised edition. To make a long story short, what we thought would be a three-month process stretched out to well over two years. We had to run off over 4,000 copies of the first mimeographed version. The present book is the final result.

The Religious Question

From the preliminary edition we received several questions about the inclusion of religious values in this manual. We think that such are valid questions and deserve an answer. Our discussion of this issue is found in Chapter 2.

The Use of the Manual

The manual was originally intended to be used as an integral part of the regular League meetings, and that remains very much a part of our teaching method. However, as unsolicited, word-of-mouth orders came in for the preliminary edition from all over the country, it became apparent that it would be used by many people who would never have the opportunity to attend the League teaching sessions. We don't think a book is an adequate substitute for personal instruction, with the opportunity to have questions answered face to face; however, in the light of its probable usage by many, we have tried to make this manual as complete and as self-contained as possible. In verbal instructions we repeat ourselves; so also in the manual, some things are said more than once where it seems appropriate for completeness.

Mutual Support

Still, a book is no substitute for people. In a society that is increasingly oriented toward contraception and abortion, many believers in natural family planning find themselves in a somewhat embattled position. Thus the League also exists to provide an opportunity for couples to share friendship, concerns, and values in an atmosphere of love and support.

Principles

As an organization, the Couple to Couple League has certain principles that guide its operation. These can be stated rather briefly with a short comment on some.

— Natural family planning is an art, and like the arts of natural childbirth or breast-feeding or swimming, it needs to be learned. In animals, for example, swimming is guided by instincts; but among men and women, the natural capacities need to be developed through learning and practicing proper techniques.

— Natural family planning is a truly humanizing art because it utilizes the human powers of observation, analysis, and interpretation. It also develops the same human strengths that are necessary for monogamous marriage and marital fidelity.

— Natural family planning is the best approach in every respect—health, morality, and in the development of married love. Natural family planning can be a marriage-building art because it requires continuous working together, cooperative decision making, and in-depth communication.

— Every couple can learn the various methods involved in natural family planning. Widespread experiments have shown that lack of education is no barrier; even the illiterate have learned to use natural family planning successfully. Present techniques are known as the "sympto-thermal" method, and scientific developments may bring about further additions to the art of natural family planning. The Couple to Couple League does not limit itself to recommending any one technique; instead, it teaches all the available techniques so that each couple can make their own decision about which ones they will use.

— Present methods can determine fertile periods accurately enough so that couples can achieve an efficiency of self-regulation that ranks with the most effective means of contraception.

— "Natural" means that which is in accord with the very being of man and woman as creatures made in the image and likeness of God.

— "Natural" does not mean "doing what comes naturally" in the sense of the easiest or most convenient. In sexual matters, associating "natural" and "easy" has unhappy results, including the contemporary acceptance of nonmarital relations and contraception.

— Couples need the help of God in placing the sexual drive at the service of authentic married love—both in respect to other men and women and in their own interpersonal relations.

— Because sexual activity is habit-forming, couples benefit from self-control and the resulting freedom that should be a part of a healthy marriage. Such self-control forms a realistic aspect of natural family planning.

— Children are a gift from God, whether asked for or not. If parents are working at becoming lovers, unplanned children will not be unwanted children but will be accepted and loved for their own sake.

— The best instruments for transmitting adequate information on natural family planning are groups of informed couples dedicated to helping other couples. Clinics staffed by professionals have been tried in various places and have not proved to be the answer. Even where successful, clinics are too limited geographically and are expensive to operate. Nor is the individual physician the general answer. Doctors are not only busy, but all too many of them simply don't know much about current natural family planning—and many of them aren't interested. Books such as this one are quite helpful to some, but they are even more helpful in conjunction with group support and discussion.

Thus, it is part of the CCL philosophy to inform interested couples through groups that have regularly scheduled meetings. Leader couples are encouraged to keep meetings small enough so that adequate discussion can take place. A series of four meetings held at monthly intervals forms the core of CCL training, and couples are requested to attend all four meetings for adequate preparation.

If you would like more information about membership in the Couple to Couple League or about starting a chapter where you live, contact CCL at the address given at the bottom of this page.

Continuing Research

Research in natural family planning is continuing, and the authors would like volunteers to help in three different types of studies. In one we want to continue to accumulate data from couples who are using natural family planning to avoid a pregnancy. A second project would involve couples who want a pregnancy. The third project is an already ongoing study of breast-feeding and natural child spacing. Participation in such studies can be helpful to others. If you would be willing to participate in any of these projects, please contact the Couple to Couple League.

Keeping Up-to-Date

The Couple to Couple League strongly encourages interested couples and other persons to keep up-to-date in natural family planning by becoming members of the League. An annual membership contribution of $10.00 provides much needed financial support to this non-profit organization. (Contributions are tax-deductible.) It also brings the *CCL NEWS* 6 times a year. Through this newsletter, the national office informs its members of any and all new developments in natural family planning as well as providing other information and articles of continuing interest. Please send checks and your complete name, address and zip code to CCL, P.O. Box 11084, Cincinnati, Ohio 45211.

1

Why Natural Family Planning?
Some Tangible Values

Introduction

It is difficult to read the newspaper for much more than a week without seeing an article on birth control. Sometimes attention is drawn to the size of the population; at other times, there is an analysis of the birth rates, which at the time of this writing have decreased to below the level of zero population growth in the United States and some other countries. Such interest in population is nothing new, whether one looks at the big world and national picture or at the small picture of the individual family size. The Reverend Thomas R. Malthus became the father of population studies with his gloomy predictions of overpopulation and starvation in *An Essay on the Principle of Population*, published in 1798, and population studies continue to be very much a part of the contemporary scene.

While many couples are concerned with the global population problems, most couples have a more urgent interest in the size of their own family. Studies have indicated that the American and Canadian family in which there is ecological breast-feeding but which practices no conscious form of family planning will have about seven or eight children.[1] That is a far cry from the dozen to fifteen children that some young couples fear they will have if they don't practice contraception from the first day of their marriage, but it is also more than many families feel they would like to manage.

In addition to the statistics that have been developed from cultures unaffected by contemporary cultural trends, the modern Western woman has encountered something that was rarely encountered by her older sisters in a culture such as rural Quebec at the turn of the century; namely, the birth of one child only ten to fourteen months after the birth of another. The fact that this is due almost entirely to the absence of ecological breast-feeding in our culture (as will be seen in Chapter 7) is unknown to most couples, and the prospect of having a baby every year is just plain scary to a great many of them.

1

This ecological imbalance was brought about by cultural pressures ("be free from your baby") and by pediatricians who led Western women to abandon breast-feeding or to become token breast-feeders at best. To attempt to deal with this situation, the obstetricians and gynecologists countered with everything that the drug companies could provide—condoms, diaphragms, foams, jellies, the Pill, the intrauterine device (IUD), and more efficient tools and techniques for abortions.

To be sure, the preceding generalizations do not apply to all doctors, and certainly the development of contraception is due to more than the absence of breast-feeding. Our point is that the emphasis by the medical practitioners concerned with the care of mothers and infants has been oriented in the recent past toward a pharmaceutical rather than a natural approach; the woman who found both a pediatrician and a gynecologist who would teach her what is recommended in this book has been a fairly rare exception to the general rule. Today, some women are fortunate enough to be able to shop around for doctors who either advocate or at least go along with the natural ways of doing things, and when they find their desired combination of pediatrician and gynecologist they consider themselves lucky indeed.

There is no denying the success of the medical-industrial complex in aiding and influencing the Western public to adopt artificial practices in both baby care and birth control. This has been costly, as we will indicate later. However, the higher the cost, whether it be in terms of dollars or health or other values, the more evident it is that any knowledgeable person today is aware that all sorts of things and services are being sold for birth control. With all these products and medical services, and with the promise of more drugs to come, why do some people sense a growing interest in *natural* family planning?

We have found that there are a number of reasons that people give for their new or renewed interest in natural family planning; these reasons tend to be of several somewhat different types. One grouping is concerned with values that are more or less tangible, material or measurable. This includes such values as ecology, esthetics, cost, effectiveness, achieving a pregnancy, physical health, reversibility, life itself, sterilization, and personal freedom. The second group centers around values that are more or less intangible or spiritual, such as self-awareness, attitudes toward a baby, personal development, personal moral authority, and religion. A third group of values is concerned with the morality both of contraception and its consequences. A fourth group of values places emphasis on marriage building. All in all, a very impressive list of values is involved in family planning. We think an analysis of these values shows that the natural ways of conception regulation are the most advantageous to the person, the couple, and to society.

In reviewing these values, it may seem to some that we are too negative toward contraception. It has been suggested that we stress only the positive values of natural family planning while not emphasizing the negative aspects of contraception. Although we are not following that suggestion, we think enough of the feeling behind it to take a few lines to explain why the subject is treated as it is. For one thing, we have found many people very concerned to learn the truth about the health and life aspects of popular contraceptive practices. Since their experience has been that the Couple to Couple League was the first place they found out some of these things, we feel it useful and perhaps necessary to provide that information, unpleasant as it may be, in this book.

Secondly, we think that some people may be reading these pages in order to get more facts for making a decision. If so, they know already that at first glance the contraceptive approach seems attractive: it is the "in" thing with most doctors, thus making it appear scientific; it looks easy; and it has the obvious feature of maximizing the possible amount of coitus, whether such maximization is a real marriage builder or not. On the other hand, they know that natural family planning requires some amount of personal self-discipline and control. However, many people, perhaps even most people, would like to know more about the various bases for comparison between the contraceptive and the natural approaches to family planning—beyond the fact that one may be easier than the other.

Thirdly, some people are interested in the philosophy behind a particular pattern of behavior. While in these few pages we cannot pursue this aspect of the question in the depth we would like to, we can at least point out some significant—and sometimes rather startling—comments made by advocates of the contraceptive approach. We assume also that this book will be read by at least a few people who are not in sympathy with the conviction that natural family planning is both the best and the only morally sound way of family planning. We would hope that as they follow some of the ideas about the philosophical and long-range implications of the contraceptive approach, they will at least come to understand that a negative stand toward contraceptive, technological birth control is not a form of longing for the past but is rather a concern that man should respond to the challenges of life in ways that are not destructive of authentic human values. It is the conviction of many that these human values are supported by the approach of natural family planning but not by the contraceptive one. Readers will have to decide for themselves whether they agree with that conviction after they have read the discussions dealing with the values that are involved in this issue.

Ecology

Some of the renewed interest in natural family planning stems from a growing realization that it is wise to live in accord with nature. Many people are appalled by the harm that has been done by men when they applied their scientific knowledge without sufficient regard for the way it would upset the balance of nature. Others are just as concerned about the bodily pollution that is caused by contraceptive drugs and intrauterine devices. As a result, there is increased concern today for doing things the natural way, whether it involves growing vegetables, feeding a baby, or family planning. It would be highly inconsistent for someone to be interested in organic foods and then to take a powerful birth control drug. It should be unthinkable that someone concerned about the life of trees or birds could be unconcerned about the life of human beings still in the womb.

We know that some people are interested in natural family planning because of their interest in the delicate ecological relationship between a mother and her nursing baby, but we don't know how much of it comes from an interest in the wider ecology movement. All we can say is that it would be consistent for ecology-minded people to be interested in natural family planning, and it would be highly inconsistent for them to criticize it.

It is also worth noting that the solutions to basic ecological problems are dependent upon the exercise of a certain amount of self-control by the human race. The acceptance of self-control as a key to the solution of the problems of physical ecology helps prepare people for the self-control that plays a part in natural family planning.

Esthetics

Esthetics has to do with the beauty or "pleasingness" of something. Natural family planning leaves the sexual embrace in its natural beauty. On the other hand, contraceptive condoms, diaphragms, foams, and jellies all have definite esthetic disadvantages. Such methods make it extremely obvious to the couple that they are interfering with the natural character of the act; they also interrupt a certain spontaneity in the couple's sexual activity. Thus, the Pill was greeted with great enthusiasm because it was a form of birth control that did away with the messiness of the applied, on-the-scene, mechanical contraceptives, and it likewise was more effective even though much more dangerous.

Cost

A quite tangible value that should not be overlooked is the almost total lack of expense connected with natural family planning. Drugs, medically prescribed devices, surgical operations, and repeated visits to the doctor are simply not part of natural family planning; the only expenses are for a thermometer, this manual, and a supply of charts. The contraceptive practice has much higher costs, and the couple who suffer some of the side effects from the drugs, devices, or surgery learn how very expensive it can be for the individual family. On a national basis, who could estimate with any accuracy the amount of money spent on the contraceptive approach—regular medical consultations, prescriptions, surgery, drugs, and devices? Could we talk in less than a billion-dollar-a-year figure?

Further financial savings are available to the couples who adopt the practice of ecological breast-feeding described in Chapter 7.

Effectiveness

A rather tangible value that everyone engaged in any form of family planning is looking for is its effectiveness. Since it is rather widely thought that only the contraceptive approaches are effective, let us state emphatically that the natural family planning system recommended in this manual is *highly* effective. Couples who were skeptical at first, sometimes very skeptical, keep telling us, "It works!"

At this point we must be a bit technical. It is standard procedure in birth control literature to express the effectiveness of any method in terms of the formula devised by Raymond Pearl in the 1930s: "x" pregnancies per 100 woman-years. The number of pregnancies is known as the "failure rate," a rather unhappy way to describe a new baby. A woman-year refers to one year in a fertile woman's life. Thus, one year for 100 women is known as 100 woman-years.

If 100 fertile women had regular intercourse for one year without any form of birth regulation or breast-feeding, the statistics indicate that 80 would become pregnant by the end of the year. The conception rate would be 80 per 100 woman-years. Methods of birth control seek to reduce the figure from 80 to something much less.

How do the various methods of birth control compare? The only practice that has a pregnancy rate of zero is complete abstinence from sexual intercourse. Every other method results in some pregnancies (or live births, if abortion be called a birth control method).

A recent review by Dr. Christopher Tietze ranked birth control methods according to their method-effectiveness.[2] This is distinguished from use-effectiveness, which can be less for every possible method. For example, if a Pill user forgets to take her Pill one day and becomes pregnant, it is not regarded as a method failure, but as a user failure. Similarly, if a couple do not follow the rules of natural family planning or make an error of judgment, and the woman becomes pregnant, it is likewise called a user failure instead of a method failure. On the other hand, if a woman on the Pill follows the rules and still becomes pregnant, it is a method failure. Likewise, if a couple follow the rules of natural family planning and the woman still becomes pregnant, it is called a method failure.

Having described the usual technical terminology, we will now make a substitution, and instead of writing "failure rates," we will refer to "surprise pregnancy rate," because when a birth regulation method fails, the result is not a *failure* but a new human being.

In the Tietze review, methods of birth control were grouped into four categories according to their effectiveness. Group A, the most effective methods, included tubal sterilization, vasectomy, oral contraceptives (the Pill), and the postovulatory basal temperature method. The surprise pregnancy rates following sterilization were in the range of .06 to .15 per 100 woman-years. The oral contraceptives had surprise pregnancy rates from .07 to .34, depending upon the type of drug. The Minipill was not in this group. Intercourse only in the postovulatory phase as determined by the basal temperature method yielded surprise pregnancy rates ranging from .0057 (a single method failure in 17,500 cycles) to .10 (5 method failures in about 5,000 cycles).

Other statistics have pointed up the variations in success or failure rate with any method and have shown the relatively high effectiveness of using the basal temperature method provided there has been adequate instruction. It is well known that motivation plays a significant role in the effectiveness of any method, particularly if using devices such as the diaphragm or condom. Needless to say, motivation is extremely important for successful natural family planning.

Tietze's Group B, highly effective methods, were less effective than those in Group A but more effective than those in Groups C and D. This group included the intrauterine devices (IUD), the diaphragm with cream or contraceptive jelly, the condom, and the Minipill. The IUD surprise pregnancy rates ranged from 1.5 to 3.0 per 100 woman-years in the first year and declined thereafter. Tietze notes that while the theoretical effectiveness of the condom and the diaphragm appears to be about the same as for the IUD, the user-effectiveness is typically on the order of 10 to 20 pregnancies per 100 woman-years.

Three significant facts should be noted about these statistics. The figures for the oral contraceptive and IUD come only from those women whose bodies can tolerate them. That is, the statistics do not take into account those women who stopped these practices because of adverse reactions. Secondly, the IUD is not a method of conception regulation but of postconception abortion, and it is quite possible that the oral "contraceptives" do likewise. (See section "Life Itself" p. 10.) For the person who respects human life from its beginning, these two methods of "birth control" are ruled out, regardless of the morality of contraception itself.

Thirdly, it should be noted that these statistics do not include the techniques of natural family planning such as observations of the cervix and cervical mucus.

In Group C, the less effective methods, were placed the various vaginal foams and jellies, calendar rhythm, and coitus interruptus.

Lastly, the Tietze report listed as Group D, the least effective methods, prolonged breast-feeding and the postcoital douche. To this we must add that most studies about breast-feeding and infertility are concerned with token breast-feeding, not the type recommended in this manual. Our own study plus the work of others indicates that there is about a 6 percent chance of a woman becoming pregnant before the return of menstruation in the first year postpartum if she is breast-feeding in the way called natural mothering or ecological in this manual.[3]

The Tietze report noted that breast-feeding infertility was very good as long as it lasted; the problem was knowing when it ended. Chapter 7 goes into this in some detail. For the present, let us simply note that the observation of cervical mucus can enable a woman to detect when ovulation is going to occur prior to the return of the first postpartum menstruation, thus further reducing that 6 percent chance of pregnancy by a factor that we cannot at this time document statistically.

G. K. Doring of the University of Munich reported a surprise pregnancy rate of 0.8 per 100 woman-years in a group following the strict temperature system and a rate of 3.1 per 100 woman-years among those having coitus up to the sixth day before the earliest previously recorded day of temperature rise as well as from the third day of elevated temperatures.[4] This is better than the rates found in the Marshall study (method failures "of 1.2 for those using respectively the post-ovulation infertile phase and 5.0 for those using the post-menstrual phase as well").[5]

A study of the Billings "mucus-only" method of fertility awareness in Tonga showed a surprise pregnancy rate of less than 2 per 100 woman-years.[6] However, this study was criticized because it did not include in its calculations the 50 pregnancies that occurred among couples who ignored the mucus sign; that is, they recognized the sign but had coitus anyway. If those pregnancies are included, the rate becomes 25 per 100 woman-years, a figure in the same category with calendar rhythm.[7]

This, of course, raises a question about the evaluation of natural methods. The natural methods provide an awareness of fertility but they do not "protect" the woman against pregnancy. If a couple is aware that coitus at a particular time will probably result in pregnancy, should that be called a "surprise pregnancy"? We think that responsible couples are looking for natural methods of fertility awareness and that, therefore, systems should be evaluated on the basis of the usable information they provide rather than on the way some couples may choose to disregard that information.

While the studies mentioned have reported on groups using either "temperature-only" or "mucus-only" methods of fertility awareness, Dr. Josef Roetzer has reported on a group using a system similar to the sympto-thermal method, a system combining observations of cervical mucus and basal temperatures. (The Couple to Couple League also includes observation of the cervix itself.) The couples in this study had coitus during the postmenstrual, relatively infertile days as well as during the postovulation, absolutely infertile phase. There were only two pregnancies, neither a "method failure," in the 3,542 cycles, yielding a surprise pregnancy rate of 0.7 per 100 woman-years.[8]

Thus, there is no doubt that among the currently available methods, natural family planning is extremely effective. Still, it is part of the philosophy of the Couple to Couple League to stress that some pregnancies are going to occur even with a pregnancy rate of less than 1 per 100 woman-years of use.

The adoption of abortion as a backstop to contraception is directly related to the absolutizing of birth control by some advocates of contraception. We believe in absolutizing only God, human life itself, and then the natural way that the Creator has given us for fertility awareness and control.

Achieving a Pregnancy

Many couples who have borne children cannot appreciate the frustration childless couples experience in their desire to bear even one child. Such couples are dismayed even more by the fact that adoption is a very slow process. Due to the vast number of abortions, couples are now waiting two or even three years before they can adopt an infant and their chance of adopting a second infant is slim. In addition, these couples can spend a great deal of money visiting specialists and going through a battery of tests due to their fertility problem.

The fertility awareness developed through the Couple to Couple League natural family planning program can be of great help to couples who have experienced difficulty or unusual delay in achieving pregnancy. In an informal survey, it was found that upwards of 80 percent of the couples attending CCL meetings to achieve a pregnancy had accomplished their objective during the course of instruction or shortly after completion of the series. To those acquainted with fertility awareness, the advice given to some couples by their medical specialists seems as futile as it is costly, and the values of natural family planning are all the more evident.

Physical Health

Physical health is an important tangible value that is respected by natural family planning. In all fairness, it can be said that it is also respected by users of the older forms of contraception, namely the condom and the diaphragm. However, such statements connot be made about the three most popular forms of birth control today: the Pill, the IUD, and sterilization. (Also, the foams sometimes cause infections.)

The same newspapers that help to promote the current contraceptive techniques also carry news about their drawbacks. Congressional hearings have been held on the medical hazards of the Pill and entire books have been written about its dangers to health. One author, Morton Mintz, in his book *The Pill,* calls it the most dangerous drug ever unleashed among the general public.[9] Although he is an advocate of contraception, Mr. Mintz condemns the Pill because it subjects women to the risk of blood clots, paralysis, and death when such risk is unnecessary. The older methods may have been less pleasing and less esthetic, but they carried no risk to the woman's health.[10] The long-term risks to health from continuous use of the Pill have yet to be determined. Not too long ago, a case of vaginal cancer was traced to the use of a drug by the patient's mother during her pregnancy about 20 years previously. Such long-term results raise all sorts of questions about the ultimate effects of using the Pill.

The intrauterine device likewise has its share of disadvantages to the health of the mother. It can cause irritation, bleeding, and even perforation of the uterus. It also seems to damage somehow the Fallopian tubes. Sometimes, the damage it causes to the uterus continues to prevent the successful carrying of a pregnancy after the IUD has been withdrawn and when the couple earnestly desire a baby.[11]

Faced with these rather obvious disadvantages to health, many couples have turned to sterilization of either the man or woman. Such a method is usually a relatively easy surgical operation that generally has a low risk to health at the time of the operation. However, sterilization of a woman by tying her Fallopian tubes has been known to result in tubal pregnancies. Such a situation is always fatal to the new life and sometimes fatal to the mother.

As male sterilization has become more popular, there have been increasing reports about various side effects. In addition to some nasty, very painful immediate reactions, there is also the problem of long-term continued discomfort.[12] A vasectomy does nothing to prevent the continued manufacture of sperm. Normally, excess sperm is discharged through a nocturnal emission, but such a natural process is prevented by a vasectomy. Thus, the sperm, a protein, has to be reabsorbed into the body's tissues; as a result, some men have experienced discomfort ranging from aching testicles to low-grade fevers. In addition, various articles have mentioned problems of psychological health suffered by some men who have had themselves sterilized. Such problems, which began only after the vasectomy, included "complete impotence, persistent premature ejaculation and even one case of vaginal irritation in one wife."[13]

Will a vasectomy improve the sexual practice and the overall marriage of the couple by relieving them from the fear of pregnancy? The evidence does not support that view.[14] Dr. William A. Nolen, writing in *McCall's,* noted that men should not have vasectomies in order to solve marital problems. "This is a trap that many couples fall into: They aren't getting along—their problems are, in part at least, related to fear of pregnancy—and they think that a vasectomy will make life wonderful again. It won't. Very few marital problems are solved so neatly. The problems that disrupt most marriages aren't cured by cutting out a bit of tissue."[15]

Reversibility

A related consideration is the permanence of sterilization. Female sterilization (tubal ligation) and male sterilization (vasectomy) are rarely reversible, and because of this, sterilization is truly a drastic step. Thus, it is out of the question for couples who simply want to space their children, and even couples who are satisfied with their present family size are counseled to consider whether they want to destroy their ability to have future children. If one spouse should die and the other should remarry, might not that couple desire another child?

A similar comment can be made about the Pill and the IUD. Sometimes they are not quickly reversible—if at all. The effect of the Pill may be long-lasting in some cases; and, as we have mentioned, if the IUD has damaged the uterus, the result may be one miscarriage after another.

On the other hand, with natural family planning there are no such drawbacks. The couple who wish to achieve a pregnancy simply begin having coitus during the fertile phase of the cycle.

Life Itself

The current, popular practice of contraception has raised the question whether the value of family planning is a value greater than life itself. Specifically, the available evidence indicates overwhelmingly that the basic mode of operation of the IUD is to prevent the seven-day-old, newly conceived human being from implanting into the walls of the uterus, thus causing its death.[16]

Thus the IUD is a method of abortion rather than conception regulation, carrying with it all the moral disvalues that accompany the killing of innocent, weak, and helpless victims. Somewhat the same thing may be said about the Pill. Drug manufacturers now admit that the Pill may act as an abortifacient (an abortion-causing drug) rather than as a means of preventing ovulation. Researchers have noted that "among women who have been followed over a considerable number of cycles, breakthrough ovulations occur in two to ten percent of cycles."[17] Since the Pill does not have surprise pregnancy rates of 2 to 10 percent, the question is raised about how it achieves its effectiveness when it does not suppress ovulation. The question is particularly acute with the low-dosage Mini-pill which may not suppress ovulation at all. Some forms of the Pill apparently affect the cervical mucus in such a way as to be hostile to sperm life and/or sperm migration, but apparently all the various forms affect the endometrium, the lining of the uterus, in such a way as to prevent implantation.

With regard to users of the IUD, the evidence allows us to say that if they are having coitus during the fertile phase of the cycle, they and their physician are in all probability responsible for the death of newly conceived children—possibly each month. We cannot make such a strong statement about users of the Pill because of the varieties of the Pill and the more confused data about how they work each month. Rather, we can repeat the statement of Dr. Albert Lorincz that it cannot be said for sure that the Pill is not acting as an abortifacient.[18] In stronger words, the evidence allows us to say that there is a definite possibility that the Pill in fact is acting as an abortifacient at least some of the time. When there are other alternatives, whether contraceptive or natural, which carry no such death-causing risks for a newly conceived human being, we fail to understand how anyone who expresses concern about the value of human life can use or prescribe the Pill for birth control. Furthermore, if it is prescribed as a drug to regulate a menstrual disorder, then it seems to us that the couple should be instructed about the possible abortifacient character of the drug and should be advised not to have coitus during the time that would normally be the fertile phase of the cycle. We are certainly not advocates of the condom or the diaphragm, but at least these are not abortifacient. Thus, they are not directly opposed to the value of life itself, however unesthetic and less effective they may be.

Sterilization: Further Considerations

Personal Freedom

Normally the topic of freedom would be grouped with the nontangible values, but some recent events have led us to consider it among the tangible values. After all, if you should be sterilized by force, would not that be a very tangible interference with your freedom? If there is a growing acceptance of having one's own self sterilized, then there is also going to be an accompanying decline in the public rejection of sterilization as something wrong or evil. People who have had themselves sterilized are usually not going to admit that they did something wrong; some of them publicly tell the world they did something good. If voluntary sterilization of oneself is no longer regarded as a moral wrong, then it is a small step in the real world (however huge a step it may be according to strict logic) to see it as not a wrong but even a good to do to someone else.

Thus, we think it is valid to be concerned that the public acceptance of sterilization may diminish the personal freedom of those who do not want to be sterilized. Certainly, we are aware that the advocates of population control through sterilization tell us that they seek only *voluntary* sterilization, but it is difficult for us to believe such talk in the face of evidence from around the world that governments have provided economic incentives for sterilization and have provided very stiff penalties for families larger than the government-approved size. For example, the sterilization programs in India have been a far cry from Gandhi's "birth control through self-control." If a body politic becomes convinced that there is nothing morally wrong with contraceptive sterilization in itself, then we can look forward to arguments such as these: "It is a social good to be sterilized; it is antisocial not to be sterilized; the government has the right and the obligation to enforce social behavior for the common good; therefore the government can impose sterilization." "Just as the government has the right to separate wage-earners from some of their money through taxation, it also has the right to separate married people from some of their fertility through sterilization." Never mind that these arguments proceed from unproved statements; logic hasn't won too many elections. The point is that when a public regards sterilization as morally permissible, it is going to be increasingly less concerned about whether it is voluntary or enforced; then, the people in a democracy will be softened up to accept arguments that equate enforced sterilization and taxation as both distasteful and unpleasant but necessary for the common good. People whose government is less than democratic may not be able to offer any counterarguments. We have the unhappy precedent that sterilization was one of the first steps taken by the Nazis to exterminate the Jews.

"Of course," many will say, "it can't happen here." The truth of the matter is that it has already begun. In the summer of 1973, the nation was alerted to the fact that certain welfare recipients were being sterilized. The particular incident that made news involved two young black girls who were sterilized with their consent, but the question of their ability to make a *meaningful* consent to a permanent loss of fertility was challenged. In this case, legal action was taken against the doctor and others, but what will happen in another decade or so if sterilization gains a stronger hold on the public mind?

We think that to avert these dangers we all need to face up to the reality of what contraceptive sterilization is all about. It is a physical mutilation of one's own body, and therefore of one's own self, by the deliberate and permanent destruction of the normal processes of fertility.

Contrary to all of this, natural family planning truly respects and builds the value of personal freedom. As we shall describe in the next chapter, it contributes to a true inner freedom, the ability to be free to say "no" as well as "yes" to one's inclinations toward coitus. How great it is to be in control of one's sexual activity rather than to feel driven by uncontrollable urges to engage in coitus or masturbation.

Psychological-Spiritual Aspects

Many find the psychological-spiritual implications of sterilization quite disturbing. Voluntary sterilization says something about the sterility of the whole person. The human person is not just a spirit encased within a body-tool through which it operates. The human being is a body-person, and what we deliberately do to our body we do to our whole self. When a person is born with a defective arm or loses an arm in an accident, we regard it as a physical imperfection and try to help him, but if a person should deliberately cut off his arm, we would judge that he suffered not just a physical imperfection but a sickness of his total person. Likewise, if a person proves to be sterile from birth, we regard it as a physical imperfection; however, when he deliberately sterilizes himself, he does something to the total person. The physical sterilization now reflects the sterility of the total person—spiritual as well as physical. It is a sign of the ultimate biologization of the sex act and a sign of a loss of hope at being able to cope with the stresses engendered by the various factors of family size, sexual urges, and socio-economic conditions. It amounts to a total admission of the inability to control one's use of sex so as to achieve effective natural conception control.

14

We realize that the preceding statements do not apply to everyone who has been sterilized. Sometimes couples have been led by their doctor to believe that this was the *only* way, at least for them. In such cases, the physician must bear much more of the responsibility than the couple themselves. In the last analysis, these physicians have dealt with their clients from a veterinary approach. Veterinarians have long been employed to eliminate surgically the fertility of our cats and dogs, but we do not think that such an approach is appropriate or humanizing for human beings. What is humanizing for men and women as made in the image and likeness of God is to understand their natural pattern of fertility and then to govern their sexual activity in accord with their desire to achieve or to avoid pregnancy. That is what natural family planning is all about.

From another point of view, deliberate sterilization offends against the commandment "Thou shalt not kill," for it involves deliberate destruction of the function of a healthy human organ. It has been a long-standing tenet of the Christian tradition that we may not destroy or mutilate healthy bodily organs of the human person. This is a reflection of the Christian recognition that the Christian does not own himself; rather, he belongs to Christ. "You must know that your body is a temple of the Holy Spirit, who is within—the Spirit you have received from God. You are not your own. You have been purchased, and at a price. So glorify God in your body" (1 Corinthians 6:19-20).

We have also heard of other disadvantages of sterilization. In some cases, as mentioned previously, it has had bad psychological effects, and in others it has created a false sense of "freedom" and an opportunity that led to infidelity.

References

[1]Nicholas J. Eastman. Editorial comments in *Obstetrical and Gynecological Survey,* 10:5 (1955), 661-662, on Gioiosa study (1955). Eastman notes that G. W. Beebe, *Conception and Fertility in the Southern Appalachians,* (Baltimore: Williams and Wilkins Co., 1942, p. 75) found a pregnancy rate of only 3 per 100 woman-years of exposure in 1,500 months of coincident lactation and amenorrhea compared with 105 per 100 woman-years in some 2,100 months outside of the time in lactation amenorrhea. Furthermore, from Canadian census figures, Eastman calculated that in rural Quebec between 1891 and 1921, when breast-feeding was common and contraception unheard of there, the woman marrying between ages 20 and 24 would average 7.9 live births. Eastman notes how close this is to the figure of 7.8 children for American wives in 1790 (Lotka, *Journal of the American Statistical Association,* 22:154 (1927).

[2]Christopher Tietze, "Ranking of Contraceptive Methods by Levels of Effectiveness," *Advances in Planned Parenthood VI,* Proceedings of the VIII Annual Meeting of the AAPPP, Boston, Mass., April 9-10, 1970, Excerpta Medica International Congress Series No. 224.

[3]John and Sheila Kippley, "The Relation Between Breast-feeding and Amenorrhea: Report of a Survey," *JOGN Nursing,* 1:4, (November-December 1972), 15-21.

[4]G. K. Doring, "The Reliability of Temperature Records as a Method of Contraception," Deutsche medizinische Wochenschrift 92 (June 9, 1967), 1055-1061. Abstracted in the *1968 Yearbook of Obstetrics and Gynecology,* p. 354. The 125 surprise pregnancies were analyzed thus in this abstract: 6 had coitus on the second day of elevated temperatures; 12 "misinterpreted temperature rises from colds, 13 conceived toward the end of the 'safe' post-menstrual period, 56 were pure patient errors and 38 had incomplete records. Conception never occurred on the third day of hyperthermia [elevated temperatures]."

[5]John Marshall, *The Infertile Period* (Baltimore: Helicon Press, 1969), p. 111. Marshall refers to the actual study, "Field Trial of the Basal-Body-Temperature Method of Regulating Births," *Lancet* 2, 8 (1968). The overall rates he observed were 6.6 (postovulation only) and 19.3 (postmenstrual as well). Eliminating the couples' mistakes, the method rates were 1.2 and 5.0, respectively.

[6]Sr. M. Cosmas Weissman, Leopino Foliaki, Evelyn L. Billings, and John J. Billings, "A Trial of the Ovulation Method of Family Planning in Tonga," *Lancet* (October 14, 1972, pp. 813-816.

[7]John Marshall, Roger Rochet, and W. Henry Mosley, "Letters to the Editor," *Lancet* (November 11, 1972), pp. 1027-1028.

[8]Joseph Roetzer, "Erweiterte Basaltemperaturmessung und Empfangnisregelung," *Archiv fur Gynakologie* 206 (1968), 195-214.

[9]Morton Mintz, *The Pill: An Alarming Report* (Boston: Beacon Press, 1970).

[10]For an inexpensive and rather comprehensive survey, see Herbert Ratner, ed., *The Medical Hazards of the Birth Control Pill.* Reprint booklet of *Child and Family* (Box 508, Oak Park, Illinois 60303). 96 pp. $1.

[11]Typical of many newspaper articles carrying criticism of the IUD was a front-page article in the *National Observer,* September 8, 1973.

[12]John J. Fried, "The Incision Decision," *Esquire* (June 1972), pp. 118 ff.

[13]Ibid., p. 120.

[14]Ibid., p. 172.

[15]William A. Nolen, "Vasectomy: A Cautionary Note," *McCalls* (June 1972), p. 136.

[16]Thomas W. Hilgers, "The Intrauterine Device: Contraceptive or Abortifacient?" *Marriage and Family Newsletter,* Vol. 5, Nos. 1, 2, 3 (January-March 1974). A slightly shorter version appeared under the same title in *Minnesota Medicine* (June 1974), 493-501.

[17]John Peel and Malcolm Potts, *Textbook of Contraceptive Practice* (New York: Cambridge University Press, 1969), p. 99.

[18]Albert Lorincz, M.D. Oral comments in a question-and-answer session at the end of his presentation on the operation of the Pill. Marriage and Family Life Workshop, St. John's University, Collegeville, Minn., June 8, 1972.

2

Why Natural Family Planning?
Some Intangible Values

Self-Awareness

Many women appreciate the self-awareness they develop in natural family planning. They are able to note physical abnormalities sooner than they would otherwise and thus can seek medical attention at an earlier date. Some women may avoid an unnecessary doctor's visit or surgery. Pregnancy tests can usually be omitted when self-awareness is developed. One woman experienced severe abdominal pain, and upon consultation a doctor scheduled her for surgery. Fortunately, she was able to contact another doctor who suspected ovulation as the cause of her agony. His diagnosis was confirmed by examination and basal temperature readings, and this woman was spared unnecessary surgery and additional hospital expenses.

Some women express a sense of satisfaction from knowing just where they are in their periodic cycle. A former user of contraception told us that whenever her period was three days late, she used to worry about being pregnant. When she started natural family planning, she was very skeptical. Within six months she became very confident. She finds she is no longer fearful when her period begins late. Once her husband teased her about this lateness. To prove that she wasn't pregnant she took her temperature reading, which had lowered. She predicted her period would begin by the following day, and it did.

Women can develop a better understanding of their bodily and emotional states through fertility awareness. A married woman writes:

> I would like to add a personal vote of thanks as a woman for bringing to me a feeling of true-self. That is, now I really seem to grasp the idea of what a cycle consists of—all the changes within me that occur. I've known this, but now all these things I don't take for granted any more. This is a very real and very deep sensation. Once again we thank you for making us aware.

A husband can also become more appreciative of the changes in moods and emotions his wife may undergo during the fertility cycle.

Attitudes Toward a Baby

Every known means of birth control results in some babies. Even women who have abortions sometimes deliver babies who refuse to die. The massive use of contraception has tended to absolutize the idea of the "wanted child" to the extent that some have recommended killing the unborn child as a backstop to contraception.[1]

The couple who use natural family planning should be conscious of the fact that they are respecting God's order of creation. With this attitude, if they should experience an unplanned pregnancy they can accept the new life as an unexpected gift from God and grow to love the child for his or her own sake. Unwanted pregnancies are usually a result of carelessness, but unwanted children are a result of lovelessness. If the sex act was an act of loving persons, then the child will be wanted and loved whether he was "planned" or not.

In a more positive vein, it frequently happens that the happy mothering attitudes engendered by proper breast-feeding stimulate a desire to have another child by the time fertility returns. This desire for another pregnancy seems to be a typical consequence of "natural" breast-feeding. It is for this reason that there is an old-time saying among nursing mothers, "Babies are contagious." This should be recognized, discussed, and decided by couples according to their particular responsibilities.

Personal Development

The practice of natural family planning requires the development of personal self-control. This is both an advantage and at the same time the biggest single disadvantage of natural family planning.

More will be said in Chapter 9 about difficulties that may arise in connection with self-control. For the present, let us simply note that it is a necessary part of personal development in every area of life. The person who has gained self-control likewise gains in self-respect; he or she also gains the respect of those who know him or her as one who has self-possession.

Sexual self-control brings about a new freedom, a freedom to refrain from or to engage in sexual relations without feeling compelled to do so because of the sexual urge. The couple who practice natural family planning in effect say to each other, "We, with the help of God, can direct and handle our emotions and instincts. We are persons who are weak but still in control. Our sexual relations are more free because they are freely chosen instead of being the result just of our urges." This doesn't involve denying that these emotions exist or calling them bad or anything of the sort. Rather, it means accepting them and deliberately placing them at the service of authentic married love. The power to do this in marriage is what has been traditionally called the power of marital purity or chastity.

Is Natural Family Planning Natural?

The mere fact that natural family planning calls for self-control and the development of skills and human potential brings up the question, "Is natural family planning natural?" Specifically, the question is raised about two aspects of natural family planning: (1) refraining from sexual relations and (2) the observation of signs and temperatures.

What do we mean by "natural" for man and woman? In the briefest terms, we mean living in accord with God's order of creation. Jews and Christians alike affirm that man and woman were created "in the image and likeness of God" and that we are called to live up to God's plan for us. Christians further affirm that one of the reasons why the Son of God became man was to teach us how to live up to the demands and potential of our human nature. In this view, God's Commandments are not *arbitrary* rules but are the rules for living up to the demands of our nature. Thus, it is not "just human nature" to lie, steal, murder, and commit various sexual sins. Common as these wrongs may be, they are offenses against the human vocation to be true to one's nature as a person created in the image and likeness of God.

This means that we believe that it is contrary to God's order of creation—and thus contrary to our nature—for married people to have sexual relations with anyone else, or to break up a true marriage and remarry, or for the unmarried to have coitus. Rather obviously, this view is not shared by all. We know that some people think that having sex with anyone at any time is really quite natural to man, and others think that it is unnatural for a man to remain faithful to one woman all his life. We could not disagree more strongly, and we would hope that those who share our convictions about sex will also agree that "natural" does not mean doing what seems easiest or most convenient with regard to sex.

When critics question whether natural family planning is "natural," they typically add that a period of refraining from genital contact doesn't fit in with their view of sexual spontaneity. This idea has been voiced so often that it has caused unnecessary difficulties for couples who would like to choose only the natural way of conception regulation. After all, if couples are led to believe that spontaneity is the key to happiness, then they are going to be prejudiced against a form of family planning that requires some restraint at certain times. Thus, because much about sexual self-control is psychological, it is important that the couple take this talk about spontaneity with a grain of salt. What is frequently meant by it is simply letting one's sexual activity be directed by his or her urges. No one in his right mind can deny the reality of these urges, but love is much more than the satisfaction of body urges. If married men and women were to be truly spontaneous according to that concept of spontaneity, we would have a lot more day-time traffic as husband (or wife) got an urge at work and sped home to celebrate it.

Several responses can be made to the question about the naturalness of not having coitus whenever the husband or wife might feel like it. In the Old Testament, the Jews were told to refrain from sexual relations for twelve days beginning with the first day of every menstruation, and everyone recognizes that there may be times in any marriage when the couple may have to refrain from sexual contact for an extended period because of physical health. Some writers have pointed up the psychological benefits to be gained from regular periods of sexual self-restraint within marriage. Thus, in answer to the question about whether it is natural to refrain from sexual relations for some time, we can surely answer that it is by no means contrary to God's order of creation to exercise sexual self-restraint, even within marriage.

Secondly, we should note that "natural" is not the same as "spontaneous." All of us know that is true with regard to sex, for we can all think of social and family needs that make it necessary to control our various sexual inclinations.

We might also note that some former users of contraceptive devices and chemicals have found that their sexual spontaneity was interfered with far more by the use of contraception. One couple put it this way after learning about natural family planning:

> We get upset with articles that say natural family planning takes the spontaneity from the marriage act. It is such a wonderful feeling to know that we are not taking the beauty out of the marriage act with an ounce of foam. Our married love has grown and become more spontaneous and beautiful than we ever thought possible.

Lastly, it should be noted that if coital spontaneity is made the guideline to happiness, parents have little to say to their teenagers whose urges and emotional needs may be much stronger than those of the parents.

With a positive approach to natural family planning, a couple can enrich their marriage through periodic self-restraint. The first rule of natural family planning is to keep on loving during times of sexual abstinence. This means finding other ways of showing mutual care and love, somewhat similar to the days of premarriage courtship. With this sort of positive approach, couples can find their marriage enriched through alternating periods of courtship and honeymoon.

A Canadian couple wrote us about their discovery of this courtship phase: "As a married couple, we are particularly enjoying the courtship phases involved in the practicing of this 'art'—they are tempting times with a tension all their own, but they bring back the rich romantic feelings of premarital days." Another couple aware of the concern among married couples that sex may become boring or dull explained that with the alternating phases "sex never gets old!"

The second question asked whether it was natural to take one's temperature, to observe the other signs of ovulation, and to keep records. What this question really asks is whether it is natural to have to make this kind of effort. Again, what we mean by natural is to be in accord with God's order of creation and not to go against His plans for us. We believe that in this sense study, practice, and hard work are natural to man. We do not think it is unnatural to spend years in study or to put in endless hours developing an athletic or artistic skill. We do not think that people who keep daily charts on their investments in the stock market or people who take their temperatures when they aren't feeling well are acting unnaturally.

Rather, in each of these cases they are developing their human potential as they use their intellectual and physical powers for a good purpose. The same is true of the practices involved in natural family planning. They are actually humanizing, since they develop and make use of the powers of observation and judgment in achieving a legitimate human goal. (This is not to say that *any* use of any human power is humanizing. The man who developed his muscles to assault or seduce another person, the person who used his brain to solve the problem of getting rid of Germany's Jews, and other such "problem solvers" certainly could not be said to be acting in a humanizing way even though they were using their natural powers.)

Personal Moral Authority

The couple who respect God's order of creation and who use only natural family planning methods can make a consistent moral stand when their teenagers begin to wonder about sex. These parents can give not only the "it might hurt someone" answers about sex before marriage; they can also explain how the sex act is meant to be a renewal of the marriage covenant. They can explain how even within marriage the partners have to exercise self-control in order to respect God's order of creation.

On the other hand, what about the couple who tell each other that their marriage will be ruined if they don't have relations for a couple of weeks even though they could still engage in other, nongenital ways of affection? It seems to us that they are on pretty thin ice when they try to tell their teenagers to postpone sexual relations for years. Young people today are quick to sense hypocrisy on the part of the older generation. Once they realize that their parents practiced contraception or were sterilized because they would not put up with any sexual abstinence, how will young people feel about any counsel their parents might give about sexual self-control? Perhaps many such parents sense the hypocrisy of preaching what they themselves refuse to practice and thus no longer say anything to their children about the need for self-control in matters of sex; perhaps that is one cause for the apparent increase in sexual activity by many young and unmarried people today.

Religion

Under the subject of "religion" there is really a twofold question. First, why did the authors include religious values in a nondenominational book? Secondly, is there a specifically religious reason for choosing the natural-methods-only approach to birth regulation?

As to the inclusion of religious considerations, we have been asked: "Why do you call CCL nondenominational when there are religious overtones in its philosophy and in this manual?" By nondenominational we do not mean nonreligious; in the same way that Alcoholics Anonymous, certainly a nondenominational organization, recognizes the presence of God, so also do we in the Couple to Couple League recognize Him. We affirm that He is the Creator of man and that He established a certain good order within creation.

To the second question, whether there is specifically religious reason for advocating natural family planning, we'll address the issue by asking: does God care?

Undoubtedly, a significant reason why many couples are interested in natural family planning is their religious conviction that contraception, sterilization, and abortion are morally wrong. Thus, in these pages concerned with the intangible or spiritual values that are involved in family planning, it may be worth-while to examine the reasons why some people have religious or faith convictions about family planning.

When we treat religion and morality in separate chapters, we are not implying that they are unrelated. Rather, we are drawing attention to the fact that religious faith itself provides a reason for calling behavior either moral or immoral particularly for those who believe that their church is guided by God. For example, if someone says he believes that coitus with somebody else's wife is the sin of adultery, he might also give as his *reason* for so believing the fact that his church teaches that way.

For him, that is the deciding reason, and he may not be able to quote any scriptural or theological reasons. In effect, he is saying that he believes that God is the ultimate author of his church's teaching and that is reason enough.

The religious issue arises with regard to family planning when some religious groups say that any attempt of family planning at all is morally unpermissible, others say natural family planning is permissible but not contraception, and others permit contraception, sterilization, and even abortion as means of family planning. An example of the first group is the Hare Krishna religion, which is reported to teach that marital coitus is morally permissible only with the intention of trying to conceive a child. The most well known representative of the second group is the Roman Catholic Church. It is less well known that the teaching of the Eastern Orthodox churches, some parts of Judaism, and of some Protestant ministers is also in this group. We think we can say that most Protestant churches allow contraception. The newspapers have made us aware that various Protestant churches have issued statements permitting abortion to alleviate various health or family problems; some allow abortion as a backstop to contraceptive failures, an attitude prevalent in Sweden.

Two comments should be noted about the Roman Catholic tradition on birth regulation. First of all, while it provides a firm and unmistakeable negative to abortion, contraception and sterilization as means of birth control, it does allow the use of natural family planning for sufficiently serious reasons. The other side of this doctrine is the positive call to generosity in the service of life according to the various circumstances of the couple. Secondly, the Catholic tradition recognizes the reality of human weakness. It therefore calls its faithful to be spiritually nourished, strengthened and cleansed for the challenge of marital chastity by frequenting the sacraments of the Eucharist and Reconciliation. It also invites its members to gain strength and insight by meditating upon the Scriptures, particularly upon the life, sufferings, and teachings of Jesus in the gospels.

A Biblical Basis

In the Christian tradition, Chapter 38 of Genesis is frequently quoted as providing a basis for the doctrine of noncontraception. Onan, the son of Judah, is obliged by the Hebrew and ancient Near Eastern custom of the Levirate to have intercourse with Tamar, the childless wife of his deceased brother. Onan, however, does not want to give her a child who will then be considered as that of Tamar and the deceased brother. Thus, he has coitus with her but withdraws before ejaculation (coitus interruptus). The text then tells us that God slew Onan because he had done a serious wrong.

Footnote interpretations of the Bible used to say that this showed that contraception was evil in the sight of God; footnotes in some modern versions typically say that Onan's offense was simply the violation of the Levirate, not the contraceptive means of doing so. We think that the modern interpretations reflect current sexual customs but fail to do justice to the entire Biblical context. First of all, in the same chapter and immediate context Judah admits that he is also guilty of violating the Levirate; and it is clear that Judah's youngest son, Shelah, is likewise guilty of the same offense. Yet neither of them is struck by God. Secondly, the punishment for violating the Levirate is well spelled out in Deuteronomy 25:5-10. The aggrieved woman may bring the offender before the elders, take a sandal off his foot, and spit in his face; then the offending brother shall be called House of the Unshod. Humiliating perhaps, but hardly the equivalent of the death of Onan.

Since the punishment for the Levirate is well-defined elsewhere in Scripture and since the father and brother of Onan were likewise guilty of violating the Levirate, an explanation which sees the sudden death of Onan simply and solely as a punishment for violating the Levirate cannot be called faithful to the context. A more adequate explanation sees his punishment corresponding to what he did (and the others did not do). He went through the motions of the act demanded by the Levirate covenant but defrauded it of its meaning; he took its pleasure but contradicted its purpose. Thus, the Genesis text can still be used as a Scriptural basis for the religious doctrine of noncontraception. This interpretation is backed up by the only incident in the New Testament where immediate death is the punishment for sin—the deaths of Ananias and Sapphire, who go through the motions of a giving act but defraud it of its meaning (Acts 5:1-11).

In the New Testament, it is possible that the Greek "pharmakeia" may refer to the birth control issue. "Pharmakeia" in general was the mixing of various potions for secret purposes, and it is known that potions were mixed in the first century A.D. to prevent or stop a pregnancy. The typical translation as "sorcery" may not reveal all of the specific practices condemned by the New Testament. In all three of the passages in which it appears, it is in a context condemning sexual immorality; two of the three passages also condemn murder (Galatians 5:19-26; Revelation 9:21, 21:8).

There is simply no doubt that the entire Biblical notion of human love points to the fact that man is called to subordinate "eros," erotic love, to "agape," self-giving love.

While not referring specifically to the issue of birth control, St. Paul's most famous discourse on love is still applicable to this discussion. It is, noteworthy that he begins and ends on the two aspects of love that are needed for the happy practice of natural family planning. "Love is always patient and kind; . . . it is always ready . . . to endure whatever comes" (1 Corinthians 13:4,7). Christian husbands are also told to love their wives as Christ loved the Church and sacrificed himself for her (Ephesians 5:25). All Christians were told by Christ on the night before his death to love one another as he loved them, a statement that has obvious overtones about selfgiving love (John 15:12). St. Paul also tells his listeners that the fruit of the Spirit is "love, joy, peace, patience, kindness, goodness, trustfulness, gentleness and self-control." He reminds them that they cannot really belong to Christ unless they "crucify all self-indulgent passions and desires" (Galatians 5:22,24).

Much more could be said about the overall meaning of the Biblical message concerning love, but the above should suffice for at least one limited purpose. It shows that it is legitimate to state that the religious doctrine of marital noncontraception has a basis in Scripture and that the practice of natural family planning with its necessity of a certain amount of sexual self-control fits well within the Christian Biblical tradition.

The Christian Tradition

A second approach to the religious question has been given by an Anglican priest, Robert Capon, in a readable book entitled *Bed and Board*.[2] Father Capon notes that it is very difficult for someone who believes that the Church is guided by the Holy Spirit to say that the Church was wrong about contraception from the first century until 1930. What he refers to is the historic fact that until 1930, all of the churches, Protestant as well Catholic and Eastern Orthodox, taught that contraception was morally wrong. The famed Connecticut laws against the sale of contraceptives were written and passed by Protestants, not Catholics.

The year 1930 is of special interest in the history of birth regulation. As mentioned earlier, in the middle and late 1920s, two medical researchers, the Japanese Dr. Kyusaku Ogino and the Austrian Dr. Hermann Knaus, working independently, discovered that ovulation occurred about two weeks prior to the next menstruation. Recognizing the possibilities of this for birth regulation, each devised a set of rules and made possible the practice of calendar rhythm by 1930. The significance of this breakthrough is seen in the fact that prior to this time it was thought that the only alternatives to a family of indefinite size were complete abstinence or contraception.

In the field of organized religion, 1930 was also a landmark year. In England, the bishops of the Anglican Church voted to allow the practice of contraception for cases of severe hardship. This was by no means a unanimous decision, and Anglican Bishop Gore warned against other moral consequences that would result. The Catholic Church through Pope Pius XI reaffirmed the traditional Christian stance against contraception, and the debate has continued to our day.

The other thing that Father Capon was referring to is the belief of Catholics, Eastern Orthodox, Anglican, and many Protestant groups, that the Church is guided in its teaching by the Holy Spirit according to the promise of Jesus at the Last Supper. Within this belief, when a doctrine is taught consistently within Christianity from the first century until the present, there is a certain presumption that such a teaching has been due to the guidance of the Holy Spirit. Father Capon was in effect asking why we should believe that the Church was wrong in its teaching about contraception for nearly 1,900 years, why we should believe that its historic teaching was not the work of the Holy Spirit. Whatever one believes on these matters, one thing is certain: Father Capon has placed his finger on the center of a religious issue that divides Christians.

A third approach might be said to take up where the second ended. Taking its cue from the words of Jesus, "By their fruits shall you know them," this approach asks what grounds we have for believing that the post-1930 advocates of contraception are giving us something that is the work of the Holy Spirit. It must be remembered that the prime religious or faith question in this matter is about which tradition is *really* the work of the Holy Spirit, the tradition of some 1,900 years that forbids contraception or the one of some forty years which either allows it or recommends it as a positive good.

Since the advocates of the contraceptive approach argue that contraception helps to sustain marriage, the critics point to two things. The most obvious is that as the practice of contraception has increased, so also has the divorce rate. Certainly there are other factors involved, but if contraception really helped to sustain and increase the values of marital communion, and if the vast majority of married couples have adopted the contraceptive approach, then the critics of that approach wonder why the unhappiness rate in marriage, as measured by the divorce rate, has increased so much—over 100 percent since 1930.[3] The increased divorce rates make it difficult to believe that contraception is the "marriage builder" it is said to be.

Several other things can also be pointed to as associated with the contraceptive movement. As we shall see in Chapter 8, one well-known writer, Walter Lippman, in 1929 blamed the use of contraceptives for the growing sexual permissiveness of his day, and the increase of premarital sex and wife-swapping in our day of widespread use of contraceptives certainly tends to support that writer's criticism.

Secondly, the matter of "who should we believe is giving us the fruit of the Holy Spirit?" has been helped by the growing popularity of abortion. A great many of the Protestant churches that issued statements accepting contraception as a means of family planning have likewise issued statements accepting abortion if contraception fails.[4] Now, the husband half of the couple who have written this book has been mildly taken to task by a well-respected Episcopal priest for inferring that such pro-abortion statements represented the thinking of the theologians of such churches. In that priest's opinion, many of these statements were heavily loaded with what he called "with-it-ness," and thus the theologians shouldn't be heavily criticized.[5]

If it is the case that the pro-abortion statements of these various Protestant churches are examples more of trying to be "with it" than of serious theological reflection, then perhaps the same needs to be said about their pronouncements on contraception. We think that most people will agree that the moral question of abortion is more obvious than the moral question of contraception. That is, most people would agree that it is easier to see that it is wrong to kill an unborn child than it is to see that it is wrong to practice contraception. Now if in this more obvious area a number of religious spokesmen have erred in saying that abortion is within Christian behavior, then we think it is rather easy to see how they could have erred in a less obvious area. Christians and Jews who understand their religious tradition know that being "with it" is no guarantee of truth. Rather, the Biblical tradition runs directly counter to that idea and raises suspicion about the desire, whether conscious or subconscious, to change doctrine in order to be more "in" with the spirit of the time.

Finally, those who criticize contraception from a religious or faith stance point to the philosophical reflections of the advocates of the contraceptive approach. (Some of these are briefly described in the Chapter 8.) When those who say that (1) contraception is religiously permissible *also* say that (2) any other form of voluntary sexual behavior is also religiously permissible, and when they say that the second statement follows logically from the first, the religious critics ask whether anyone really has grounds for saying either statement reflects the work of the Spirit.

In summary, the question of religion or religious moral authority in the contraception issue is really the question of which side the authority of God is on. For those who believe that God has revealed Himself in history (the traditional belief of Jews and Christians) and that the Holy Spirit has guided the Church of the New Testament from Pentecost until the present at least in its major teaching, the constant tradition for nineteen centuries against contraception provides a powerful argument. The moral decline and the increased divorce rates that have paralleled the acceptance of contraception, the acceptance of abortion by many of the religious spokesmen who accepted contraception, and the statements of some that they cannot say "no" to any voluntary sexual acts once they have said "yes" to contraception—all of these provide further support for those who cannot agree that the acceptance of contraception by the modern Western world has been the work of the Holy Spirit.

Natural family planning, on the other hand, does not run contrary to the teachings of any major religion, although it may not be acceptable to groups that teach that procreation must be sought at each coital embrace. Furthermore, as we have seen, natural family planning frequently involves a significant group of attitudes—respect for one's body and healthy, respect for each other, respect for the order of creation, respect for life, and the winning of sexual freedom through self-control and the grace of God. All of this is so much in keeping with the Biblical tradition of Jews and Christians that even those who are not disposed to agree that natural family planning is the *only* way might say, from a religious point of view, that it certainly is by far the *best* way of family planning and that it is at least the moral norm.

References

[1]A rather notable example: Richard S. Unsworth, et al., *Sexuality and the Human Community: A Task Force Study Document.* (Philadelphia: General Assembly of the United Presbyterian Church in the U.S.A., August 1970), pp. 26-27.

[2]Robert Farrar Capon, *Bed and Board: Plain Talk About Marriage* (New York: Simon and Schuster, 1965), p. 87.

[3]In 1930 there were 1.6 divorces per 1,000 population and in 1970, 3.5 divorces per 1,000 population, an increase of 119 percent. Marriages during the same time increased from 9.2 to 10.7 per 1,000, an increase of only 16 percent. From *Statistical Abstract of the U.S.,* 1972, p. 50.

[4]The task force report cited in Note 1 above was indicative and typical of other statements by various Protestant church bodies.

[5]For example, a Methodist pro-abortion statement was issued without the consultation of that church's known and respected theologians, including Prof. Paul Ramsey, who is known for his pro-life stance. There is also increasing evidence that other pro-abortion statements purporting to represent a church's official view on abortion in fact have only represented the view of the individual spokesman or committee. Perhaps in time the same thing will be said about the pro-contraceptive statements made a few years back, thus enabling such churches to return more easily to the historic Christian tradition.

3

The Basic Physiology Of Human Reproduction

The Man's Part

The man's part in human reproduction is relatively simple compared with that of the woman. The testicles, which are contained in a sac called the scrotum, manufacture sperm on a regular basis. The prostate gland produces a fluid that combines with the sperm and is called semen. When the man is sexually excited, his penis stiffens so that it can be inserted into his wife's vagina. When he is sufficiently stimulated, an ejaculation occurs which expels the semen into his wife's vagina.

Millions of sperm may be deposited in any act of sexual intercourse. It takes only one of those sperm to join with his wife's egg (ovum) to create a new life. Under the microscope each sperm looks like a tadpole with a headlike body and a "tail." The tail thrashes around and enables the sperm to swim upward in the woman's reproductive channels to meet the egg. If an egg is present, the woman is fertile and one of the sperm may penetrate it. If the sperm and the egg unite, a new human life begins. This process is called *conception*. (It is also known as the process of fertilization; see fig. 3.1).

If an egg is not available, conception cannot occur even if sperm are present. Instead, they will simply disintegrate within a short time. The length of sperm life after ejaculation in the vagina varies according to conditions in the woman's reproductive channels, especially the vagina. Ordinarily, sperm life after ejaculation is short. If there is no cervical mucus in the vaginal tract, sperm life is anywhere from 1/2 hour to 24 hours, depending on the acidity of the vaginal tract. In the presence of cervical mucus, sperm life is usually 72 hours (3 full days) at most, but under some conditions sperm may live for as long as 6 days.

A man reaches biological sexual maturity during his teens, sometimes even earlier. The growth of hair in the armpits, on the face, and in the area around and above his penis indicates this new biological power. However, in contrast with his biological sex, the young man's inner sexual maturity is by no means automatic, nor will he always progress in

29

maturity. In his behavioral life, he may be more immature at age twenty-four, even sinfully immature in a sexual exploitation of others, than at age fourteen. In short, the young man typically has a struggle of many years to keep his biological power at the service of authentic love.

It should be noted that once the normal biological sexual power has developed within a young man, he is capable of fathering a child at any time. In contrast, a woman is fertile only a few days each month.

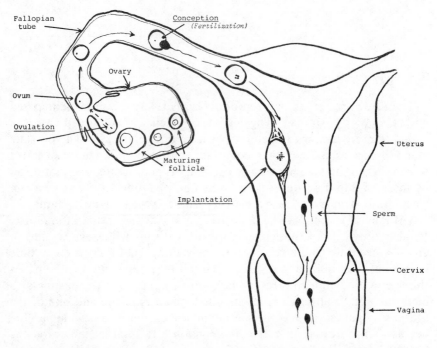

Figure 3.1: The Process of Becoming Pregnant

The Woman's Part

The woman's part is considerably more complex than the man's. A normal man possesses a relatively simple reproductive system and continuous fertility; a woman has a much more elaborate reproductive system that gives her a rhythmic cycle of fertility and infertility. She undergoes certain hormonal changes each month that may affect her both physically and emotionally. An understanding of these changes is necessary for successful natural family planning.

There are six body parts or organs that will be mentioned regularly in discussing the woman's role in becoming pregnant. In this chapter we will describe the bodily changes and signs related to fertility for which these organs are responsible.

The Ovaries

Ovary is the name given to each of the organs that act as the store-houses of all the eggs (ova) the woman will ever have (see fig. 3.2). A woman has two ovaries, one on each side of the uterus. Within the ovary each ovum has its own container, called a *follicle*. Once a young woman has reached a certain level of biological sexual maturity, one of these follicles ripens and ejects an ovum approximately every month except during pregnancy and for a variable time after childbirth. (This latter time may be considerable during ecological breast-feeding, as will be explained in Chapter 7.)

The process by which an ovum is released from its follicle is called *ovulation*. After ovulation the ovum lives from 15 to 24 hours. The range of life makes it apparent that ovum survival is not the same for all women. During this time, the ovum may join with a sperm to begin a new human life. If it does not join with a sperm, the ovum begins to disintegrate and is no longer capable of fertilization.

After ovulation, the follicle that released the egg has a new role to play and gets a new name. It is now called the *corpus luteum,* and its function is to send out a chemical signal, a hormone called progesterone. This hormone is emitted after ovulation for about 10 to 14 days and has three effects that interest us: it keeps the lining of the uterus intact; it prevents another ovulation from occurring; and it causes the basal body temperature to rise. When the corpus luteum ceases to produce progesterone, the lining of the uterus breaks down and is sloughed off during *menstruation*. The time between ovulation and menstruation is usually about two weeks, with a normal range of 10 to 16 days.

The Fallopian Tubes

Next to each ovary is a tube called the Fallopian tube that connects to the uterus. When an ovum is released from the ovary, it is picked up by the tube and begins to travel toward the uterus. Conception takes place in one of the Fallopian tubes when a sperm cell has come up the tube and united with the ovum.

The Uterus

Within this organ, sometimes called the womb, the baby develops. The uterus is normally about the size of a small pear, but it stretches many times that size to accommodate the growth of the baby. Each month a lining called the *endometrium* builds up inside the uterus. The purpose of this lining is to provide a place for the newly conceived life to implant itself and to give it nourishment. If conception takes place, then the lining remains during the entire pregnancy.

If conception has not taken place, about two weeks after ovulation this lining will begin to disintegrate and will be passed out of the woman's body. This process of sloughing is sometimes called the monthly "bleeding," although the woman is not really bleeding in the same sense as from a cut. More technically, this process is called menstruation. It is also called menses because it usually occurs once a month and the Latin word for month is "mensis."

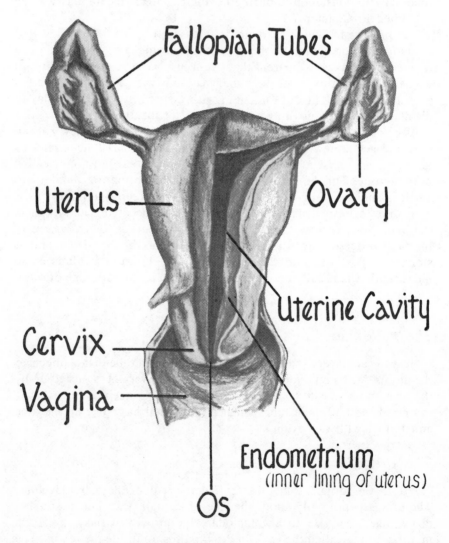

Figure 3.2: The Female Reproductive Organs

The Cervix

The cervix is a channel about an inch in length that joins the body of the uterus to the vagina. The lower end of the cervix has an opening called the *os* (the Latin word for mouth). The cervix and the os can be felt by a finger inserted into the vagina. The os undergoes certain physical changes around the time of ovulation. During childbirth, the cervix opens wide to allow passage of the baby from the uterus into the vagina. Lining the cervix are glands that secrete mucus under the stimulus of the hormone estrogen.

The Vagina

The vagina is the female sexual organ that receives the male penis. As mentioned before, sperm deposited in the vagina enter the cervix, if it is open, then progress upward through the uterus and into the Fallopian tubes, where conception may take place.

The Breasts

The mammary glands or breasts are likewise part of the woman's overall reproductive physiology even though they are not directly involved in the process of uniting sperm and ovum. During the process of breast-feeding, the sucking stimulation at the breast, through a complicated hormonal interaction, suppresses ovulation and hence fertility for a variable length of time (see Chapter 7).

The Menstrual Cycle

Once a girl reaches a certain stage of biological sexual maturity, she begins to have a regular cycle of ovulation and menstruation. In some girls, this begins as early as age ten, and most are experiencing it by age fourteen. This process normally continues well into a woman's forties and sometimes into her early fifties. However, in the later years she is much less fertile for a number of reasons. Toward the end of her years of fertility, a woman enters stages called premenopause and menopause, the latter frequently called the change of life. During this time ovulation and menstruation may become irregular, and eventually they cease completely. The actual cessation of all menstruation is called menopause. Popular usage tends to group premenopause and menopause under the latter term.

On the average, most women menstruate about every 28 days. This is an average figure and should not be applied to any individual case. Some women regularly have shorter cycles of 25 or 26 days or less;

34

others may have cycles up to 40 days or more. *Almost all women* vary somewhat from their own average. For example, Mrs. A may have an *average* cycle length of 28 days. A cycle range of 5 days is well within normal variation. Therefore, it would not be unusual for Mrs. A to have some cycles of 26 and others of 30 days. This degree of variation is not considered irregular. Some women, however, may have cycles ranging from 25 to 50 or more days, and these rare cases are considered irregular.

Regardless of the length of the cycle, a woman is fertile for only a few days in each cycle. These days occur about 10 to 16 days *before* the beginning of the next menstruation. For an individual woman, the interval between ovulation and the following menstruation is usually very regular (see fig. 3.3). Mrs. A may have 12 days while Mrs. B has 15 days, but Mrs. A will usually not vary much from her own 12-day pattern. An exception is frequently found in the first few ovulatory cycles after pregnancy, when the interval between ovulation and the next menstruation is usually relatively short.

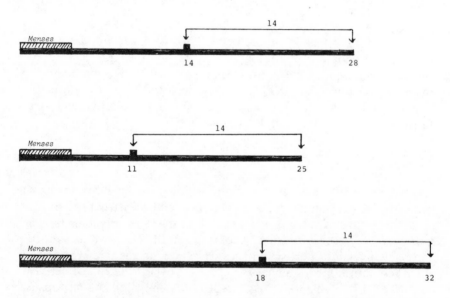

Figure 3.3: The Regularity of the Post Ovulation Phase

The top diagram in fig. 3.4 shows a typical menstrual cycle. If a woman is not pregnant or lactating abundantly, she has these recurring cycles. After one menstrual period, the lining (endometrium) of the uterus begins to build up. Then she ovulates. If she doesn't conceive, the endometrium is discarded and menstruation occurs. That is what creates the menstrual bleeding, and the cycle is under way again.

The Fertility Cycle

The menstrual cycle is also a fertility cycle. During each cycle there are three phases related to fertility: (1) the relatively infertile phase, (2) the fertile phase, and (3) the absolutely infertile phase (see fig. 3.4, lower diagram).

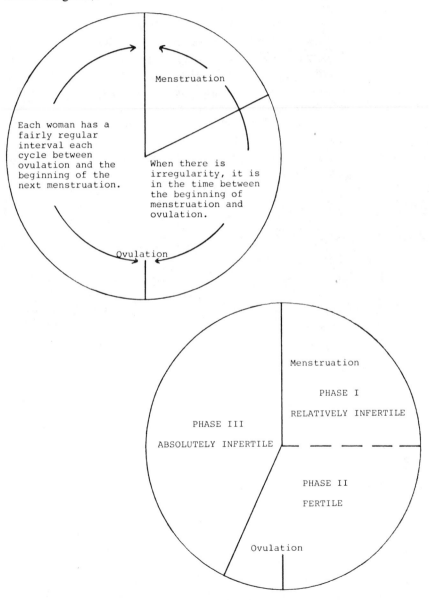

Figure 3.4: The Menstrual-Fertility Cycle

Phase I

The relatively infertile phase begins as the menstrual flow decreases. It is an extremely rare situation for conception to occur during the first few days of heavy menstrual flow, but once the flow begins to decrease, conception is a possibility. Thus, the interval between the beginning of decreased menstrual flow and the beginning of the absolutely infertile stage must be regarded as relatively infertile or as fertile.

Within the cycle, the length of the relatively infertile phase varies the most. That is, for the woman who has irregular cycles, it is the length of Phase I, the relatively infertile phase, that will vary from cycle to cycle. (The woman who *regularly* has a short cycle may be experiencing either a short Phase I, a short Phase III, or both.)

Within this relatively infertile phase, days that are closer to ovulation are more likely to be fertile than the earlier ones. Part of the art of natural family planning is for each couple to learn enough about the wife's pattern of cycles to make intelligent decisions about which days in this phase may be relatively fertile or relatively infertile.

Phase II

The fertile phase consists of a relatively few days in each cycle. If sperm life is three days and the life of an ovum is two days, then there are only five days in that cycle on which coitus or genital contact can result in pregnancy. However, in natural family planning, days of safety are normally added at both ends of the most fertile days to take into account an early ovulation or a double ovulation within twenty four hours of the first one.

One sign that the fertile phase has begun is the appearance of preovulation cervical mucus, but for some women the fertile phase may begin before the first observable sign of cervical mucus. That is, enough mucus may be present for fertility before the woman actually is able to observe it. A sure sign that the fertile phase has ended is a basal temperature thermal shift that has been sustained for the third morning reading. (These terms will be explained in chapter 4.)

Phase III

The absolutely infertile phase begins a few days after ovulation and lasts into the fast flow days of the next menstruation. Because ovulation has occurred several days previously, conception is no longer possible, and thus this phase is called the absolutely infertile phase or the phase of postovulation infertility.

There are three signs that the postovulation, absolutely infertile phase has begun:

(a.) the basal temperature thermal shift for three days;

(b.) the drying up and absence of mucus into the fourth day past the qualitative peak of the mucus symptom; and

(c.) the closing, firming up, and lowering of the cervix for several days after its peak of openness, softness and elevation.

All of these are explained in Chapter 4.

4

The Signs of Ovulation

In this chapter we describe the major observable signs that accompany ovulation and then interrelate these signs in a typical example. The major signs of mucus, cervical changes, and temperature rise are due to changes in certain hormone levels, so first we should have a brief review of the role that these hormones play in the fertile menstrual cycle.

A hormone is a chemical substance secreted by one of the body's endocrine glands that affects some other bodily function. The process of ovulation begins when the pituitary gland (located near the base of the brain) secretes a hormone called follicle-stimulating-hormone—FSH (see fig. 4.1). This FSH then stimulates the development of a follicle and the ovum it contains in one of the ovaries. The stimulated ovarian follicle then secretes another hormone, called estrogen. The estrogen causes the glands lining the cervix to produce mucus and to undergo some other changes. About a day prior to ovulation, the output of estrogen reaches a peak (see fig. 4.2). At peak estrogen output, a second pituitary hormone, called luteinizing hormone—LH—is produced, which stimulates the ovarian follicle to ovulate.

After ovulation, the follicle is called the corpus luteum and begins to secrete progesterone. As mentioned in Chapter 3, the progesterone prevents another ovulation from occurring in that cycle; it also causes the basal body temperature

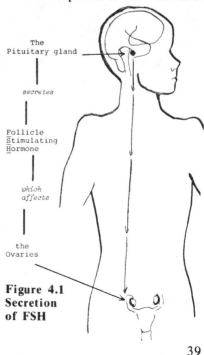

The Pituitary gland

secretes

Follicle Stimulating Hormone

which affects

the Ovaries

**Figure 4.1
Secretion
of FSH**

40

to rise and the cervical mucus to thicken and form a plug in the cervical canal. The phase of the menstrual cycle under the influence of the corpus luteum is called the luteal phase.

The signs of ovulation will be described in the order in which they occur within a woman's menstrual cycle.

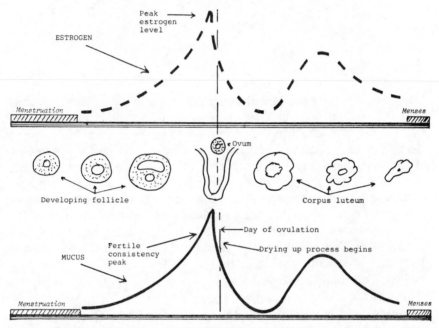

Figure 4.2: Estrogen Levels and Typical Mucus Pattern

Sign 1—Cervical Mucus

Because a secretion of cervical mucus always precedes ovulation, it is a valuable sign in the art of natural family planning. However, it is not yet known whether all women, even when properly informed, can always recognize the mucus when it first appears. There are four things to remember about cervical mucus.

1. It provides a favorable environment in which sperm can live. Under ideal mucus conditions, it may be possible for sperm to live beyond the ordinary life span of 72 hours. In the absence of mucus or with adverse mucus conditions, sperm may live only a few hours. However, couples practicing natural family planning should not plan on a shortened sperm life.

2. It provides a stream, so to speak, in which the sperm can swim up the cervical canal and eventually reach the Fallopian tubes to unite with an ovum.

3. It is present prior to ovulation as nature's way of assisting conception.

4. It changes in quality both before and after ovulation and generally disappears a few days after ovulation.

A short time before ovulation, the cervix reacts to the increase in estrogen and begins to secrete mucus into the vagina. The duration of this mucus discharge may vary from one to several days; four to six days is fairly typical. At first, if obtained on the fingertips, the mucus is rather cloudy and tacky or it breaks as soon as any effort is made to stretch it. It might be compared to the mucus that you blow from your nose in the last stages of a cold. As ovulation approaches, the mucus usually becomes more plentiful and, more important, at the same time it becomes stretchy and clear in appearance, much like raw egg white. It may stretch one to six inches, and it becomes slippery and tenacious. This is the type of mucus that indicates the time of greatest fertility, and it may last from one to several days.[1] Of greater importance, this mucus also causes a feeling of wetness or lubrication on the outer lips (labia) of the vagina.

As long as the mucus has *any* of the characteristics of being clear, stretchy, slippery and/or providing a feeling of wetness, it is to be considered the fertile type of mucus. This mucus is usually clearer than at other times, but it may be cloudy, tinged with blood, or brown or yellow as well.

Somewhere around the day of ovulation, the mucus begins to change again in quality. It loses its qualities of being like clear or cloudy raw egg white, stretchy, slippery and "wet". It becomes non-stretchy and tacky, thicker, more opaque, and then it usually disappears. In this manual, the *drying up process* refers to the days of distinctly changed tacky mucus that come after the fertile type mucus and before the completely dry days.

The *peak mucus day* is very simply the last day of the fertile type mucus before the drying up process starts. When the fertile type mucus lasts for several days, the **last** day is the peak day. **This usually does not coincide with a peak in the quantity of the mucus; the peak in quantity typically occurs 1 or 2 days before the peak in quality.**

Ovulation frequently occurs on the first day of the drying up process. However, sometimes ovulation comes before the peak mucus day and it has likewise occurred as much as 3 days after the peak mucus day.[2]

The most important thing about the mucus sign as an indicator of infertility is its distinct change and/or disappearance after it had the characteristics of the fertile type mucus. *Thus for purposes of determining the beginning of Phase III, the "dry" or the "drying up" days are the important ones.*

Observing the Sign

Women who understand what is happening recognize a feeling of wetness between the external lips of the vagina during the days of mucus. Sometimes they describe this as a distinct feeling of wetness, of lubrication, or of slipperiness, while on other days they notice a distinct feeling of dryness. This feeling of vaginal wetness is very important because it may reveal the presence of the mucus sign when it cannot be noticed by other means. For some women, wetness or slipperiness provides the only indication of the presence of mucus.

The majority of women can observe the mucus when wiping with toilet paper, by the vaginal feeling and/or by visual observation of the mucus on the paper. Some women may get the mucus they need to test its color and stretchability from what has been discharged onto their underwear. Another way to test for mucus is to insert a finger into the vagina. Although this may sound distasteful to some, it should be recognized that this doesn't differ much from the insertion of a tampon-type sanitary napkin. The internal type of observation may be the most reliable with certain women; some women have noted the fertile-type mucus with an internal examination when no "external" mucus could be observed. With others, internal examination may be helpful until they learn to observe the mucus externally.

A correspondent suggested the use of a tampon for women who have difficulty in noticing the mucus. Inserted for several hours, it allows the mucus to accumulate on it. This apparently makes the observation of the quality much easier in some cases. A friend of our correspondent found this helpful because she was having great difficulty noticing mucus otherwise. We have not researched this, and we do not recommend it as a general practice. However, since it may be helpful in an occasional case, we pass it on for whatever it may be worth.

The difficulty is the learning process. While learning, it is recommended that the woman write down any observation for mucus at the end of the day. Once this observation is learned, it is an easy process and the woman begins to notice or feel the difference automatically without having to remember to check. The most important point is that the woman learn to recognize this pre-ovulation sign; how or what method she uses is immaterial as long as she learns to make the observation.

The observation is made **periodically throughout** the day and recorded at night. However, sexual intercourse at night may obscure mucus observations the next day. The residue and vaginal secretions that result from intercourse may make it seem that there is ovulation mucus when there is not.

Experienced women have noted that the mucus discharge is not constant throughout the day. Thus it is very important that this observation be made *periodically* during the day. Any observations of wetness or other characteristics of fertile mucus make it a "wet" day. The toilet-paper observation provides a convenient, periodic test for some; other experienced women report a sensation of wetness without having to make specific external or internal tests.

Some women notice a mucus discharge every day. However, most and perhaps all of these women can learn to distinguish the difference in their own types of mucus upon close observation and with experience.

Mucus of varying quality may occur after ovulation, but this need not concern the woman if the basal temperatures and the presence of the dry days have assured her that ovulation has occurred. If a second ovulation should occur, it would take place within twenty-four hours of the first one.[3]

Practical Use

The mucus sign can be used most of the time to determine the transition from the relatively infertile phase into the fertile phase and then the transition from the fertile phase into the absolutely infertile phase.

1. The Pre-ovulation Mucus Sign of Fertility

As soon as the menstrual flow begins to lighten or has ceased, the woman should begin to observe the mucus sign. Couples wishing to avoid pregnancy should not have sexual intercourse or genital contact from the time when mucus appears until the beginning of Phase III. It should be remembered that the mucus provides an environment that keeps sperm alive. Cases have been reported where sexual intercourse six days prior to the estimated time of ovulation has resulted in pregnancy. That would be quite unusual, but it points up the fact that under certain mucus conditions sperm can be long-lived.

The possibility of not detecting mucus in time is probably increased when there is a relatively short mucus patch, e.g., less than 6 days counting the days from its appearance through the first day of drying up. Thus other rules for pre-ovulation fertility awareness have been developed. (See Chapter 6.)

Pregnancy can likewise result from intercourse using mechanical contraceptives (diaphragm or condom) or from coitus interruptus during the fertile phase. Thus, these should not be used. If a couple should choose to have such contraceptive intercourse, they are obviously not practicing natural family planning; and any surprise pregnancies must be attributed to the contraceptive method, not to the sympto-thermal method.

2. Determining the Day of the Peak Mucus Symptom

For the purpose of determining the beginning of the absolutely infertile phase, it is the drying up or disappearance of the mucus that is significant. The day before the drying-up process begins is the last day of cervical mucus that is like raw egg white in its consistency or that produces the feeling of vaginal lubrication or wetness. This is the day that is called the day of the peak mucus symptom even when there are several days of practically identical mucus signs. Thus, the peak mucus symptom day is known only by hindsight. For example, Mrs. A noticed the clear stretchy mucus on Tuesday and Wednesday. Then on Thursday, she noticed that it was tacky and opaque, and she no longer had the feeling of vaginal wetness. She would then label Wednesday as the peak day.

3. The Mucus-Only Rule of Thumb

It has been determined that the fourth day past the day of the peak mucus sign usually coincides with the third day of elevated basal temperatures. Thus, the following rule of thumb has been developed for determining the beginning of Phase III according to the mucus symptom taken by itself alone:

"Beginning of Phase III = Peak Mucus Day + 4." Alternatively: "Beginning of Phase III = Fourth day of Drying Up."

If Wednesday was the peak day, then Sunday would be the day indicated by this rule of thumb as the beginning of Phase III.

However, as mentioned above, sometimes ovulation comes as much as three days past the day identified as the peak day of mucus. Thus, a couple using the mucus-only rule of thumb of "Peak + 4" might have coitus on the day after ovulation, a day of possible fertility. Accordingly, the mucus-only rule of thumb needs to be modified for greater accuracy in determining the beginning of the absolutely infertile period.

4. The Sympto-thermal Rule of Thumb

The sympto-thermal method refers to a system of fertility awareness that combines the observations of mucus, cervix, basal temperatures, and other secondary signs in putting the theory into practical judgments. In this system, the various signs corroborate one another. Thus, its rule of thumb for determining the beginning of Phase III with the mucus sign ordinarily would be as follows:

"Beginning of Phase III = Peak Mucus Day + 4 *provided there is sufficient basal temperature corroboration.*"

The meaning of the italicized phrase will become more clear when the basal temperature sign of ovulation is explained later in this chapter and when the various signs are combined for interpretation in Chapter 6.

Sign 2—Changes in the Cervix

The second sign of ovulation is a change that takes place in the cervix. The cervix is the part of the uterus that opens into the vagina—the opening which becomes part of the birth canal during childbirth. It is firm and cylindrical and about one inch thick. The opening of the cervix, the os or mouth, feels like a little depression or hollow in the center.

During the infertile phases of the cycle, the cervix remains firm and is easy to reach. As ovulation approaches, the following changes take place (see fig. 4.3):

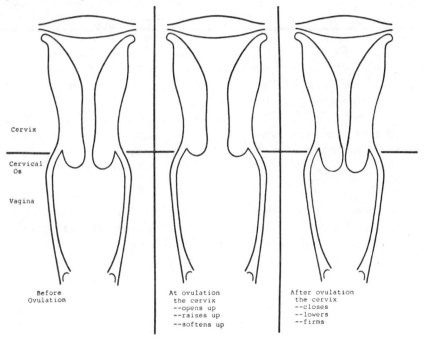

Figure 4.3: Changes in the Cervix

1. The os opens up (dilates) enough to accept a fingertip.
2. The portion of the cervix protruding into the vagina becomes softer, attaining a rubberiness and softness similar to the walls of the vagina.
3. The cervix rises and becomes more difficult to reach.
4. There is an abundance of mucus.
5. The mucus makes the cervix feel more slippery.

These signs appear gradually and it takes several months to recognize them and become experienced in their interpretation.

After ovulation, the cervix soon changes back to the way it was before ovulation:

1. The os closes, frequently more tightly than it was before its pre-ovulation opening.

2. The whole cervix becomes firmer; the tip becomes like the tip of the nose.

3. The cervix moves lower; it becomes easier to reach, and it frequently becomes lower than it was before its pre-ovulation rise.

4. The mucus changes in quality or consistency and is difficult to obtain.

5. The absence of mucus makes the cervix feel drier in comparison with its feeling during the peak of mucus.

Some people believe that these changes in the cervix are the most positive signs of ovulation. However, everyone recognizes that it takes *practice* to detect these signs, which are not as easily measured as the basal temperatures. The changes in the cervix are in terms of several comparisons—more open or closed, higher or lower, softer or firmer, more slippery or drier. Thus we stress that the woman observe these changes throughout several cycles.

The writings of Dr. Edward F. Keefe,[4] which we have found so helpful on this subject, suggest that a woman who examines her cervix through three cycles should be able to recognize the changing signs.

Observing the Sign

The changes in the cervical os can be observed by the woman herself chiefly through examination by touch. (A doctor can detect the opening of the os visually with a special instrument.) One way for the woman to do this is to put one foot up on a low chair while standing on the other foot; while in this position she inserts the index or the middle finger or both up the vaginal tract to touch the cervix. Pressing down on the abdomen with the other hand frequently makes it easier to touch the cervix. Another way is to make this observation while sitting on the toilet. Some women find this latter method makes it easier to reach the cervix. Because this sitting method of observation may make the cervix seem lower and easier to reach, it is very important that the observation be made in the same way each time. Otherwise, the woman may confuse differences in the ease of reaching the cervix with changes in the actual position of the cervix itself. Some may also find that the cervix is partially dilated after a bowel movement, and this would be unrelated to ovulation. In such cases the woman would check this observation at another time during the day. The observation of the cervix can be made at any time of the day or night, but it needs to be done every day during the time before and after ovulation in order to notice the changes that are taking place.

Furthermore, some experienced women have noticed that the opening of the cervix seems to vary on a cyclical basis each day, being higher in the morning after a night's rest and lower later in the day. Therefore, the woman should choose a fairly consistent time for making this observation, preferably after having been up for some time. (In the rest of this book, the changes in the cervix are generally referred to in terms of opening and closing instead of mentioning the raising-lowering and softer-firmer characteristics as well. This is done for the sake of writing convenience and is not intended to lessen the importance of these changes. In fact, the characteristic of the cervix being high and sometimes unreachable is perhaps the easiest and most frequently made observation among experienced women. Thus, "closing" is frequently used as a general term to describe all three of the fertility changes in the cervix.)

A woman who is first learning how to detect this sign should do this every day of the cycle for the first three months. In that time she will most likely become experienced in detecting the changes she is looking for, and she can then reduce the number of days on which she makes this observation. Women who are experienced with this method can actually detect the os closing within an afternoon or day. Some women use this method exclusively to detect the occurrence of ovulation. However, the Couple to Couple League generally recommends that a woman should confirm that ovulation has taken place through the rise in the basal temperature or through the mucus observations, or both.

Practical Use

The changes in the os are very closely related to the cervical mucus and the practical import is the same. When the os begins to open up and rise, it is a sign that ovulation is near. If a couple wish not to have a pregnancy, they should refrain from coitus or genital contact during this phase. Once the os has closed, the couple should wait at least three days for safety. The rule of thumb can be stated thus:

"Beginning of Phase III = Day of Cervix Closing + 3." Alternatively: "Beginning of Phase III = Fourth Day of the Closing of the Cervix."

For greatest effectiveness, this rule of thumb ordinarily should be used with the basal temperatures. Thus the sympto-thermal rule of thumb for the cervix would be as follows:

"Beginning of Phase III = Day of Cervix Closing + 3 *provided there is sufficient corroboration from the basal temperature pattern.*"

Experience with this fertility sign is a real asset to the nursing mother and the woman approaching menopause. Both the cervix observation and the mucus observation are valuable to the woman who finds it difficult to interpret temperature recordings or who experiences extreme irregularity.

Some possibly helpful hints

Now that both the mucus and cervix symptoms have been described, two comments may be helpful.

1. The Keefe method of mucus observation. Edward F. Keefe, M.D., the New York gynecologist who has been assisting women with the sympto-thermal method for some 25 years, suggests the following method of mucus observation:

Insert two fingers through the vaginal tract to the cervix. Place them on opposite sides of the cervix and gently but firmly "milk" the cervix. This should squeeze out a sample of the mucus within the cervix if any is available. Keep the two fingers together as you withdraw them. Separate and check for stretchiness, etc.

Some women have reported that this method enables them to detect cervical mucus a day before they have felt it on the lips of the vulva; others have reported that this method made their entire mucus observation more certain.

2. Finding the cervix. Sometimes a woman seems unable to find her cervix at first. In some instances, the husband has been able to help. He makes the observation and tells her its approximate location, height, and description. Then once she finds it the first time, she typically can find it by herself thereafter.

Sign 3—Ovulation Pain

When the ovum is expelled from the ovary, it breaks through a thin membrane that covers its follicle container. Frequently, a surface blood vessel is broken by this breakthrough and bleeding occurs. The lining of the body cavity is very sensitive to internal bleeding, and its reaction results in pain. This pain is technically called "mittelschmerz," meaning pain in the middle, although it is usually felt on one side or the other in the general vicinity of one of the ovaries. Sometimes, it lasts a few hours; at other times, it may last for one or two days, depending on the amount and duration of the bleeding. For some the pain is negligible, but women have been known to experience great discomfort, even to the point of being doubled over with pain.

Observing the Sign

Some women never feel this pain, but many others feel it every month. Many women have noticed this ovulation pain for years but never knew what it was. Once they know, they can recognize it and associate it with ovulation.

We cannot say for sure whether ovulation pain is a sign that ovulation is about to occur, is occurring right now, or has just recently occurred.

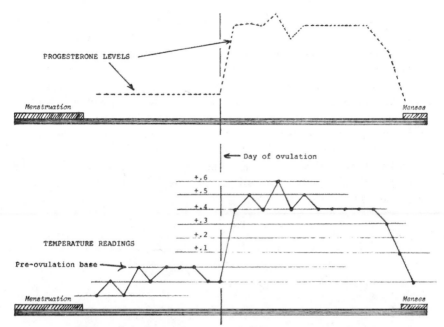

Figure 4:4: Progesterone and Temperature Levels

The membrane-breaking bleeding may take place when ovulation is just starting, and it may take a day or so for the ovum to break through the membrane of the follicle.

Practical Use

Even though the ovulation pain doesn't exactly pinpoint the time of ovulation, it may help a woman determine its approximate day. It is useful strictly as a secondary sign that helps to confirm the other signs.

Couple to Couple League policy is to recommend that a couple should not rely on the ovulation pain as a primary means of detecting ovulation. For one thing, it might be confused with minor intestinal pains or cramps, and if it occurred during sleep, it might not be 'felt at all. The signs of the mucus, cervix, and basal temperature are far more reliable.

Sign 4—Temperature Rise

As soon as the ovarian follicle has ejected its ovum, it begins a new function. It becomes the corpus luteum and begins to release progesterone. This hormone causes a woman's basal body temperature to rise slightly, usually about 5/10 of a degree—for example, from 97.7° to 98.2° (see fig. 4.4).

A person's basal body temperature is the temperature of the body at rest, uninfluenced by food or drink or activity. It rises and falls in a cyclic pattern throughout the day and night, with the lowest point being in the morning than it is later in the day. Normally, it continues to rise after a person's regular wake-up time and rises about 1/10 of a degree every half hour until it reaches the normal high base, which is around 98.6°. Both the rate of rise of 1/10 of a degree per half hour and the 98.6° temperature are averages and may not hold true in any individual case.

Ovulation is followed by a sustained rise in temperature called the *thermal shift*. The new level will usually be 4/10 to 6/10 of a degree

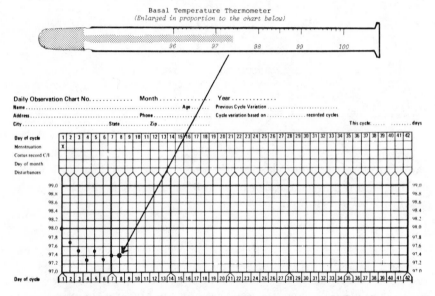

Figure 4.5: Basal Temperature Thermometer and Graph

higher than the *pre-ovulation base*. The pre-ovulation base is established by the normal high temperatures on the six days preceding the beginning of the postovulation rise in temperature. When the basal temperature has been elevated 4/10 to 6/10 of a degree above the pre-ovulation base for at least three consecutive days, a definite thermal shift has been established, and it is certain that ovulation has occurred.

Observing the Sign

To observe the rise in her basal body temperature, a woman should take her temperature when she awakens in the morning. Because her basal temperature will rise if she stays in bed, she should take it for five minutes at the same time each morning. However, it is not necessary to record immediately, and if she chooses to stay in bed for a couple of hours, she may just set the thermometer aside in a safe, dry place and return to sleep. (However, she should never place it where it would be subject to additional heat — on top of a radiator or in front of a hot air vent.)

Is a special thermometer needed? It is helpful but not absolutely necessary. A special basal body thermometer records only within the range of 96° to 100° and is very accurate. It is also more readable than the typical sickroom thermometer (see fig. 4.5).

How should a woman take her temperature—orally, rectally, or vaginally? Rectal and vaginal temperatures tend to be more accurate than oral temperatures because oral temperature readings can be affected by insufficient mouth moisture, having one's mouth open, etc. Many people who teach natural family planning recommend using only the rectal or vaginal method. However, the experience of those associated with the Couple to Couple League is that most women can obtain satisfactory temperature recordings by taking the temperature orally. If temperatures taken orally tend to be irregular, then a woman should use one of the other methods. The basal temperatures of the vagina and rectum will record a little higher than those of the mouth. Therefore, a woman should not vary her method of temperature-taking during any given cycle. Those who take their temperature rectally or vaginally do not need to insert the thermometer very deeply, and they must be careful not to break it while it is thus inserted.

Does a woman have to remain in bed while taking her temperature? Rather obviously, this question applies only to those taking their temperature orally. The experience of the Couple to Couple League is that most women can get accurate oral temperatures even if they do not remain in bed. Therefore, a woman can spend her five minutes of temperature-taking in bed, or she can get up with the thermometer in her mouth and perform light morning duties such as going to the bathroom and getting dressed. Such light activity will not affect the temperature pattern, but it is advisable to have a uniform practice of either staying in bed or getting up. She may test this practice simply by recording her temperature at the end of five minutes in bed, shaking the mercury down, rising as mentioned above, and checking the temperature again after five minutes of such light activity. After a few mornings of this, she can see for herself whether her temperature has been raised by this light activity or has remained the same.

Three cautions:
1. A woman who takes her temperature orally should never have a drink of any kind or a cigarette before taking the temperature. On the other hand, common sense tells us that a glass of water at 4:30 A.M.

isn't going to affect an oral temperature reading at 6:30 A.M.

2. A woman who gets up while she is taking her temperature should be careful. We have known of women who have broken thermometers while brushing their hair.

3. A woman should not fall asleep while taking her temperature.

A common question: Does getting up during the night affect the morning basal temperature? Usually this question has reference to taking care of a child during the night, and the amount of actual activity is negligible. This will not significantly affect the morning basal temperature. Even when the woman is up for quite some time during the night, her morning basal temperature will usually be quite normal if she has been able to get a good hour's sleep before taking her temperature. If the temperature should be unexpectedly elevated after a night of interruptions, a notation of the disturbance should be made on the chart.

When and how should the temperature be recorded, and who should do it? Once the temperature has been taken for five minutes, either the woman or her husband may record it. The authors of this manual recommend giving the recording job to the husband as his part if their team approach. It is a good practice, but not absolutely necessary, to record it immediately on the temperature graph (see fig. 4.5). If that isn't practical, a notation can be made in a notebook, etc. If no notation is made, then be sure to keep the thermometer away from any heat until a recording is made. The mercury won't go down unless it is shaken down, but it might go up if subjected to heat.

After the temperature has been recorded, the reading and recording should be rechecked, and then the thermometer should be shaken down so that it is ready for the next day.

Two notes of caution:

1. Do not shake down the thermometer in the bathroom or kitchen. There are too many hard things around to hit it on and break it. The best practice is to shake it down over your mattress. Thus, if it should slip, it would likely hit some soft blankets instead of a hard floor or sink. Hold on to the thermometer firmly, even on the upstroke.

2. A theremometer is a delicate instrument, the basal thermometer more so. If you wash it, do so *only with cold water*. (A basal temperature thermometer may rise too high in the presence of a fever; the mercury may separate, and it may be impossible to shake it down properly. A woman suspecting she has a fever over 100 should use a regular clinical thermometer.)

Interpreting the Temperatures

The important thing about the basal temperature sign is that after ovulation the temperatures will remain elevated. The rise has to be sustained at this higher level to be reliable as a sign that ovulation took place.

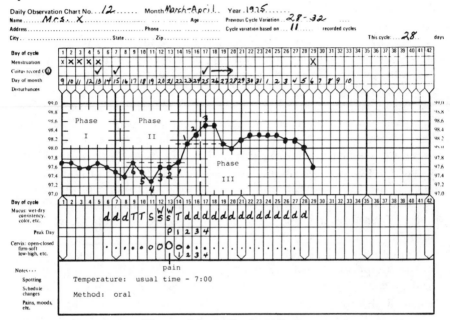

Figure 4.6: A Typical Cycle

Fig. 4.6 shows a typical cycle with an easily observed thermal shift. Note that the day of the cycle is given in the top line, and the first day of menstruation is day 1. All the temperatures for the first 14 days are either *at* or *below* 97.7° in this example. They begin to rise on days 15, 16, and 17 and hold there on day 18, showing a distinct thermal shift. Note also that the new level is distinctly higher than the pre-ovulation level. The change in temperature level is usually 4/10 to 6/10 of a degree. Sometimes, it is more; sometimes, very infrequently, it is less. Part of the *art* of natural family planning is that the couple learn to recognize what is normal for a particular woman.

In this illustrated case the first day of rise (15) was 4/10 of a degree above the pre-ovulation high level of 97.7°; then there followed temperatures showing a rise of 6/10 and 8/10 of a degree above that level.

The dip on days 19 and 20 is not really typical, but it is not at all unusual either. Note that it remained above the pre-ovulation high level even though on day 20 it fell to only 3/10 of a degree above that level.

Practical Use

1. *Temperature-only method.* For years many couples have been using basal temperatures alone to determine the beginning of the absolutely infertile period, with the following rule of thumb:

"Beginning of Phase III = third day of thermal shift," the thermal shift being indicated by temperatures 4/10 to 6/10 of a degree above the pre-ovulation high levels.

In cases where the woman cannot make (or chooses not to make) the mucus and/or cervix observations, the basal-temperature-only system still can be successful. However, ordinarily this system has been superseded by the sympto-thermal method.

2. *Sympto-thermal method.* The mucus and cervix signs can be of great help in the interpretation of the temperature pattern. These other signs of ovulation can make it evident that the rise in temperatures is due to the postovulation progesterone and not some other cause. Thus, in the sympto-thermal method the thermal shift is determined by a temperature rise that has been preceded by the appearance of the mucus sign and is accompanied by the drying up and/or disappearance of the mucus. Therefore, the rule of thumb emphasizing the temperatures is as follows:

"Beginning of Phase III = third day of a thermal shift accompanied by the disappearance of the mucus and/or cervix signs of fertility."

Once again, the thermal shift ordinarily requires a basal temperature rise of at least 4/10 of a degree above the pre-ovulation high level.

The best proven test of the beginning of the absolutely infertile phase is a clear thermal shift of at least three days accompanied by the disappearance of the mucus signs that had previously indicated fertility. Sexual relations may be resumed on the evening of the third day of such sustained basal temperature elevations with confidence of being in Phase III. An additional margin of safety can be gained by waiting until the fourth day of sustained temperature rise. Such a practice can also provide psychological reassurance, but it is not necessary as a general rule for natural family planning.

Other Signs

Some women will experience other signs that will indicate the period of greatest fertility. Dr. Prem notes that these signs include "increased libido, abdominal bloating, ovulation pain (mittelschmerz), vulvar swelling and slight bloody staining. These usually occur simultaneously with mucorrhea just prior to the temperature rise."[5]

The woman who has these or any other particular signs should note them on her charts. If they occur regularly, they may prove to be very helpful in determining the time of ovulation.

Putting It Together (Fig. 4.6)

For the sake of simplicity, let us assume that Mrs. X is a woman of normal fertility. She has a regular cycle of 28 to 32 days, and she menstruates regularly about the fifteenth day after ovulation. As soon as the menstrual flow has ceased, about day 5, Mrs. X begins making an examination for mucus. Typically she won't find any for several days. By day 9 Mrs. X begins to notice cervical mucus that is tacky and nonstretchy. On day 12 it seems to reach a peak in clearness, it stretches several inches, and she has a distinct feeling of vaginal wetness.

On day 13, Mrs. X feels a pain in her abdomen that she associates with ovulation. Her cervix has risen and is open enough to admit the tip of her finger. By day 14, the mucus has become tacky, and the feeling of wetness has gone; her cervix has begun to close. On day 15, her temperature has risen at least 4/10 of a degree and on days 16 and 17 it remains high, her cervix is closed, and the mucus has disappeared. Thus, on day 17 Mr. and Mrs. X may resume sexual relations with the assurance that Mrs. X has passed the fertile stage of her cycle. (In Chapter 6 we also provide an example showing the best timing to *achieve* pregnancy.)

What about sexual relations during the relatively infertile period prior to the pre-ovulation mucus? If we assume that Mrs. X has sufficient records to state that her cycle is never shorter than 28 days, then the application of the 21-day rule (explained in Chapter 5) would mean that day 7 is the last day in Phase I on which she would have sexual relations or genital contact.

More examples are provided in chapters 6 and 10.

The Debate About the Mucus Sign

Because the mucus sign can indicate the beginning of fertility, the peak of fertility, and the beginning of postovulation infertility, it has been suggested by some that natural family planning use this sign alone without reference to cervix and basal temperature signs that are also indicators of fertility and infertility. This mucus-only approach has been stressed by the Australian physician Dr. John Billings, who prefers to call it the "ovulation method." However, since all methods of natural family planning are ways of determining the approximate time of ovulation, other people call it the "Billings approach" or the "mucus-only-method." We will use the latter term.

The Couple to Couple League recognizes the distinct contributions to the science and art of natural family planning that are made by the mucus sign. It is invaluable during the time following childbirth and during the period of premenopause, and it is of great help for most situations of severe irregularity. Nevertheless, the League is not prepared to recommend the mucus-only method as the best or only method of natural family planning. First of all, it is the philosophy of the Couple to Couple League to instruct couples in *all* the methods of natural family planning and to recommend the use of a combined system. However, a couple may choose to use one sign only, and that is their own choice to make. Secondly, the mucus-only method has not been tested extensively enough to be endorsed without reservation by the Couple to Couple League. Thirdly, there are some cases in which we do not believe that the mucus-only method is particularly helpful. Some of these will become evident as we explain the system.

Rules for the Mucus-Only System

1. During menstruation and any vaginal bleeding, do not have coitus or genital contact. The reasons for this are twofold. First, the menstrual flow obscures the mucus sign. Secondly, sometimes a bloody discharge or spotting occurs at or about the time of ovulation, and since the mucus-only system does not provide the positive assurance of ovulation that is provided by the basal temperature, this method has to caution against coitus during any bloody discharge or spotting. That is, in the mucus-only method, a woman does not know if a bloody discharge is a light menstruation or a spotting due to ovulation.

2. Immediately after menstruation, begin making the mucus observation. (This should also be done under the combined system.)

3. The dry days after menstruation are available for coitus as days of Phase I relative infertility.

4. During the time between menstruation and the appearance of mucus, do not have coitus on successive days. The reason for this is that the residue from intercourse on one evening may be still present the next day and obscure the mucus observation. Again, a woman might observe the mucus but *thinks* it was just the seminal discharge, thus thinking she was still quite infertile when her fertile phase may have actually begun.

5. Once the pre-ovulation mucus has appeared, refrain from coitus and genital contact until the fourth dry day past the day of peak mucus.

6. If fertile-type mucus should appear again during the cycle, treat it just as the first mucus period: refrain from coitus until the fourth dry day past the last day of the fertile-type mucus.

7. In all of this, we repeat that the woman should remember that the mucus sign is frequently observed just by noticing the lubricative feeling of vaginal wetness. Secondly, the quality or consistency of the mucus is much more important than the quantity. (See also pp. 74 to 77 for further comment about the detection of mucus.)

Some Questions and Answers

Does the mucus-only system actually provide more days available for intercourse than other methods of natural family planning?

It all depends upon the comparison and the cycle length; all the variation comes in the pre-ovulation phases. For short-and average-length cycles, the basal temperature with the 21-day rule provides more days for intercourse since it allows coitus in the menstruation period, and this is not allowed under the mucus-only system. On the other hand, where there is a cycle variation of 28 to 40 days or more, the days allowed with the 21-day rule remain constant even in the longer cycles, while the mucus-only system provides more relatively safe days. The maximum number of relatively safe days is discussed under a "relaxed-combined system" described in Chapter 10.

Can every woman use the mucus-only system?

The experience of women associated with the Couple to Couple League indicates that as high as 15 to 20 percent of women have difficulty in observing the mucus. Some say they cannot find any at all. This may be due to a complete absence of mucus (and possibly an infertility problem) or the presence of a relatively small amount, or it may be due to inexperience. On the other hand, some women indicate that they notice mucus continuously. Even though most of these women learn to distinguish the special qualities of the mucus that comes before ovulation, we believe that a definite cutoff day in the relatively infertile period is still helpful and sometimes necessary.

If a woman observes mucus continuously, can she use the mucus-only system?

It seems to us that this is one of the real problems associated with the mucus-only system. Many, perhaps most, women learn to distinguish the fertile mucus from the ordinary mucus they experience continuously. However, they will usually need to relate the mucus sign to the basal temperatures in order to become familiar with the changes in mucus consistency. Furthermore, during some cycles, even the relatively experienced woman who has a continuous mucus discharge may become confused and have difficulty determining the first appearance of the pre-ovulation mucus.

In cases where the woman has difficulty in determining the beginning of the fertile-type mucus because of a continuous mucus discharge, the mucus-only system would call for continence not only during the menstruation period but also until the fourth day past the peak day, assuming the woman could distinguish the peak day. In such cases, the combined system using a 21-day rule for determining the end of Phase I, the basal temperatures, and perhaps also the cervix and the mucus sign is clearly superior to the mucus-only method.

Does the mucus-only system provide positive proof that ovulation has actually occurred?

No. Only the elevated basal temperatures provide positive proof that ovulation *has* occurred. Rather, the mucus generally indicates the time immediately *prior* to ovulation. It is a possible though an infrequent occurrence to observe the mucus sign without a subsequent ovulation even when a woman is having regular cycles. The cycle may be anovulatory (without ovulation), or a second phase of mucus may indicate ovulation later in the cycle. Therefore, it is important that users of the mucus-only approach continue to be aware of any development of a second period of mucus and to regard it as pre-ovulatory and fertile. This obviously necessitates daily observations, a good idea whether following the mucus-only or the combined system. Basal temperature observers would be alerted about such an anovulatory first phase of mucus by the absence of the required thermal shift.

Does the peak mucus sympton always come a full day before ovulation?

No. According to research done with twenty-two women and reported by Dr. Billings, ovulation, as determined by hormonal tests, occurred about twenty-two hours after the peak mucus symptom *on the average.* However, in one case ovulation occurred two days before the peak symptom; but, more seriously, in others it occurred as late as three days after the peak symptom.[6] Using the rule "Peak Mucus + 4," a couple thus might have coitus only one day after the first ovulation, and coitus at such a short interval after ovulation would have a definite possibility of producing pregnancy. On the other hand, the basal body temperatures do not become elevated until *after* ovulation, thus providing positive assurance that ovulation has occurred. In the combined (or sympto-thermal) method of fertility awareness, the basal temperatures provide a check on the mucus sign, and the mucus sign helps to interpret the temperatures.

For these and other reasons, we in the Couple to Couple League continue to think that natural family planning normally should include a 21-day rule and basal temperature records for the greatest effectiveness. Thus, we see the practical use of the cervical mucus as follows:

1. Its presence and subsequent drying up provide an excellent check on basal temperatures. This is particularly useful where the temperature rise is somewhat ambiguous. The fourth day past the peak of mucus will normally coincide with the third day of a sustained temperature elevation.

2. Among the vast majority of women who are able to observe accurately the pre-ovulation mucus, it takes on a special significance in

three cases because it provides a sign of impending ovulation: (1) the lactating mother if she ovulates before her first postpartum menstruation (see Chapter 7 on breast-feeding), (2) the woman who has serious irregularity during the childbearing years, and (3) the woman who has the irregularity frequently associated with the premenopausal period.

Until further research clears up some questions about the cases mentioned above and others, the Couple to Couple League will continue to recommend an approach that combines observations of mucus, the cervix, and basal temperatures. However, we know from experience that some women who start out on a combined system decide to rely primarily on one or another sign, sometimes mucus alone or in combination with the cervix, sometimes primarily the cervix sign, and sometimes primarily or exclusively the basal temperatures. This is not at all opposed to the Couple to Couple League's teaching philosophy, which is to instruct couples about all the natural signs and then let them choose the combination that they find the most helpful.

References

[1]E. L. Billings, J. J. Billings, J. B. Brown, and H. G. Burger, "Symptoms and Hormonal Changes Accompanying Ovulation," *Lancet* (February 5, 1972), pp. 282-284.

[2]Ibid., p. 283.

[3]W. M. Moore, "Ovulation Symptoms and Avoidance of Conception," *Lancet* (March 11, 1972), p. 588. Dr. Moore notes that there is no solid evidence of a second ovulation occurring several days after the first one.

[4]Edward F. Keefe, "Self-Observation of the Cervix to Distinguish Days of Possible Fertility," *Bulletin of the Sloane Hospital for Women*, Vol. VIII, No. 4 (December 1962), pp. 129-136.

[5]Konald A. Prem, "Temperature Method in the Practice of Rhythm," *Child and Family* (Fall 1968), p. 313.

[6]Billings, op. cit., p. 283.

5

Charting

Good charting makes interpretation both easier and more accurate. Therefore, we emphasize the value of complete and accurate records. The chart in fig. 5.1 is used by the Couple to Couple League and was designed to include the information we think is important. Once a person becomes familiar with it, it is simple to understand and to use properly. (Charts may be purchased from the League; write to us at the address given in the Acknowledgment of this book).

Daily Observation
Chart No. _____ Month _____ Year _____
Name_____ Age_____
Address _____ Phone_____
City _____ State _____ Zip _____

Daily Observation Chart No. _ _ _ _

When you first start using this particular form of chart, place a "1" in this space, and add one for each succeeding cycle. This may seem arbitrary, but such uniform notation will be helpful when charts are presented to counselors for help in interpretation.

Month and Year

Write in the time covered by this particular cycle. Frequently a menstrual cycle will overlap two months; then be sure to write in both months, for example, November—December. Write in the year, which may seem so obvious at the time as to be unnecessary, but if someone else is looking at it later, it will be quite necessary. Again, if this cycle overlaps December and January, be sure to write in both years, e.g., "*Month* December-January; *Year* 1974-1975.

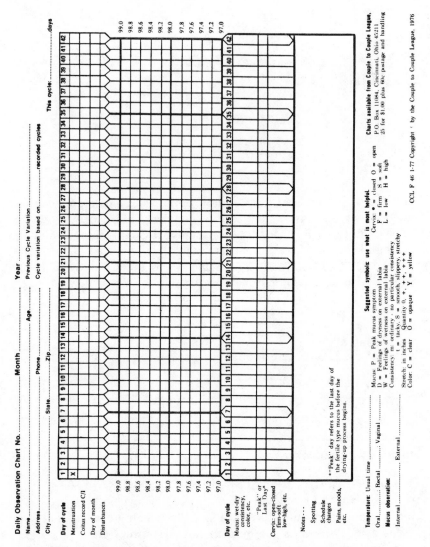

Figure 5.1: Sympto-thermal Daily Observation Chart

Name, Address, etc.

All this information is important when charts are submitted to the Couple to Couple League teachers or other counselors.

Attention is called to the value of recording your telephone number on any chart submitted to the Couple to Couple League or other counselors. CCL teaching couples are instructed to review the charts handed in at meetings and to call the couple if the charting seems to indicate some lack of understanding. For example, one couple told us they understood the method perfectly and were using it to postpone pregnancy; yet their chart showed coitus during the fertile period. A quick telephone check revealed that they had turned the system backwards and were abstaining during the infertile time and having coitus during the fertile period. (By some chance, the woman did not become pregnant in that cycle.) When people have coitus is their own business, but if they have come to the Couple to Couple League to learn when coitus will not result in pregnancy, then we would like them to understand the method correctly. Thus, we have this policy of reviewing the charts of couples attending our meetings.

If your instruction is solely through this manual, you may send us your charts for review. If you do so, please note if you will accept a collect phone call, or send a self-addressed stamped envelope. It will also be important for you to provide the coitus record, and you should indicate *your* judgments about the dividing lines between Phase I, II, and III.

Previous Cycle Variation . . . .

Cycle variation based on . . . . recorded cycles

This cycle: . . . . days

Previous Cycle Variation

This refers to the range of previously recorded cycle lengths. For example, if you have records showing that your shortest cycle was 28 days and your longest cycle was 34 days, you would record "28-34" in this space. If another cycle is either shorter or longer than the previous variation, then you change the "cycle variation" figures accordingly.

Cycle Variation Based on _____ *Recorded Cycles*

In this space, you record the number of cycles that are included in the "Previous Cycle Variation." Do you have only three recorded cycles on which to base this range? Then write down "3" in this space. Do you have records of two years of cycles? Then write down the appropriate number of cycles, which will probably be between 24 and 27.

If you have been keeping records on some chart or form other than this one, use those records in determining the *previous cycle variation* and the *number of cycles on which that variation is based.* Thus on *Daily Observation Chart No. "1,"* there could be a *Previous Cycle Variation* of *"28-34" based on "17" recorded cycles,* etc.

64

This cycle: _____ *Days*

This space is for recording the length of the cycle on this chart. A cycle begins with the first day of menstruation and ends on the last day before the next menstruation. The figure placed here should tie in with the recording on the *Menstruation* line below.

Day of cycle	1	2	3	4	5	6	7	8	9	10	11	12	13	14
Menstruation	X													
Coitus record C/I														
Day of month														
Disturbances														

Day of Cycle

Day 1 is the first day of menstruation. The chart provides for 42 cycle days; for longer cycles, another chart should be used and the numbers .changed. Always start a new chart with the beginning of a new menstruation.

Menstruation

An "X" is placed in the square for each day of menstruation. The first "X" has been prerecorded on the chart; write an "X" for the rest of the days of the menstrual flow. In addition, record an "X" on *this* chart for the first day of the *next* menstrual period. For example, if the next period begins on what would have been day 37 of this cycle, record an "X" on day 37. This indicates that the present cycle has been 36 days long.

Then record a "36" for *This cycle:* _____ *days* in this example:

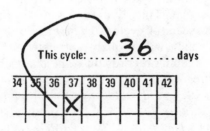

Coitus Record C/I

On your own charts, indicate every instance of coitus. This is so that if a surprise pregnancy should occur, a counselor can help you to understand why.

On the other hand, some couples may not like putting such information on a chart to be handed in to a teaching couple. However, for a teaching couple to know whether a learning couple understands the sympto-thermal method, it is necessary that they know what the learning couple regard as the limits of the fertile period. Thus, such charts should include two things:

1. A definite indication of the *intellectual* judgment about where the fertile period began and ended. Draw a line between Phases I and II and another between Phases II and III.

2. An indication of at least the *last 2* occasions of coitus (if any) of the pre-ovulation, relatively infertile period and the *first* coitus during the postovulation, absolutely infertile period. Also record any coitus in Phase II.

The *C/I* after *Coitus record* refers to "Complete" or "Incomplete." If the chart has a record of every coitus during that cycle, then the "C" should be circled. If the *Coitus record* line on a chart has omitted any recordings of coitus, then it is incomplete, and the "I" should be circled.

Day of Month

This line is to be filled in beginning with the first day of menstruation. If menstruation begins before midnight of a given day, then that day is placed in the same column as Cycle Day 1. If menstruation begins after midnight, then the date of the new day is placed in the column for Cycle Day 1. We find it handy to draw a slash mark ahead of time through the calendar dates for the Saturdays and Sundays.

Disturbances

This line is for making any sort of disturbance that might affect the basal temperature recordings. For example, several drinks on the night before might affect the basal temperature the next morning. A sore throat or a cold might raise it slightly. A fever certainly will affect the temperature readings. If you forget to set the alarm and don't take your temperature at the regular time, then take it when you awake, *but also* mark the disturbance column and write in the actual time in the "Notes" section below.

Such recording of disturbances helps to isolate temperatures that are high or low because of reasons having nothing to do with the fertility hormone levels, and interpretation is thus made easier and more accurate.

The Temperature Graph

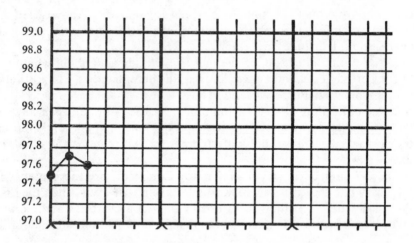

The heavy dark line on the left is day 1, and the other heavy vertical lines occur at weekly intervals—days 7, 14, 21, 28, 35, and 42.

The horizontal lines indicate the temperature levels; each line represents a difference of 2/10 of a degree from the next line.

Make your recordings on the vertical lines. For readings that fall between the 2/10 lines, make your recording halfway between the lines. For example, in the illustration above, the reading for day 1 is 97.5°, for day 2 it is 97.7°, and for day 3 it is 97.6°. If a reading is between 97.5° and 97.6°, pick the lower number; in this example, it would be 97.5°.

Day of Cycle

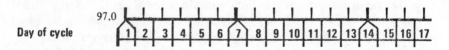

The *Day of cycle* line below the temperature graph is identical to the one above it; it is provided simply for easy reference.

Mucus Notations

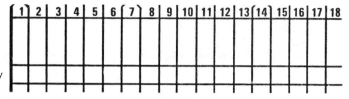

Mucus: P = Peak mucus symptom
D = Feelings of dryness on external labia
W = Feelings of wetness on external labia
Consistency: m: ordinary - no particular consistency
t = tacky, S = smooth, slippery, stretchy
Stretch: in inches   Quantity O, +, + +, + + +
Color: C = clear   O = opaque   Y = yellow

Beginning with the end of menstruation, make the proper notation *each day* in the proper space. Use the symbols that you find most helpful, but try to be as definite as you can in your use of the symbols. For example, "T," "S," and "W" provide more precise descriptions than the "M" symbol, which is best used to describe that mucus that some women seem to have all the time. If there is no mucus or feeling of vaginal wetness, *be sure* to mark the "D" for dryness. If you do not put down a notation for every day, then you won't know what your mucus pattern was for that cycle. Since the disappearance of mucus is important, it is necessary to record the "dry days" after ovulation.

Peak Day

Place a "P" in the space for the day of peak mucus and then number the following spaces 1, 2, 3, and 4 for the four days of drying up. Remember that you cannot determine the peak of mucus until the next day when the mucus symptom has changed. Where there is more than one day of the peak type of clear, stretchy, wet mucus, regard only the last day as the peak.

Mucus observation:

Internal _____External _____

Place a checkmark in the place for the method or methods you are using for mucus observation. If you are making internal observations, remember that you will always notice some wetness inside the vagina. This should not be confused with the external feelings of wetness on the lips of the vulva (the entrance to the vagina) which feelings help to indicate the presence of the more fertile type mucus.

Cervix Notations

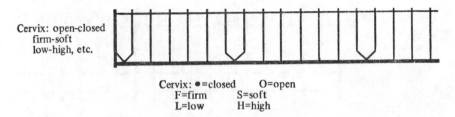

Cervix: open-closed
firm-soft
low-high, etc.

Cervix: ●=closed   O=open
F=firm   S=soft
L=low   H=high

Some women find one form of cervix notation more helpful than another; some will want to use only one feature for notation; others may want to use more. The most important thing is to be consistent in your method of recording. For the open-closed notation, use circles of varying sizes ranging from a dot to one that is as wide as the daily observation space. Use the initials "F" and "S" to note firm or soft, and the initials "L" and "H" to note low and high. Remember that the cervix opens up, softens, and rises to prepare for ovulation and then follows a reverse pattern after ovulation.

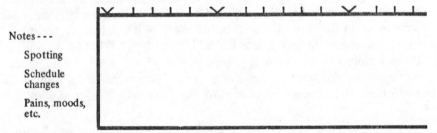

Notes - - -

Spotting

Schedule changes

Pains, moods, etc.

The blank space for notes should be used for writing down explanations for any "disturbances" marked above as well as for jotting down anything else that may be helpful in understanding or learning the fertility pattern.

Temperature: Usual time _

Oral _ _ _ _ _ _ _ ; Rectal _ _ _ _ _ _ _ _ ; Vaginal _ _ _ _ _ _ _

Temperature

Write down the usual time at which the basal temperature is taken, and check off the method of taking it—oral, rectal, or vaginal. Remember that rectal and vaginal temperatures may give more consistent readings than those taken orally and that the vagina is usually more germ-free than the mouth. This last point is made to alleviate any qualms about being unsanitary if the vaginal method is used.

The most important thing about temperature recordings is consistency. Take the temperature *at the same time* each day. If you change this method of taking your temperature, do it at the beginning of a cycle, because rectal and vaginal temperatures will be a little higher than oral temperatures. If you should change during a cycle, *be sure* to note the changed method.

Other Notations

21 Day Rule

It is recommended by the Couple to Couple League that couples have coitus only during Phase III, the absolutely infertile period, during the first six months of natural family planning practice. The purpose of this recommendation is to give the woman ample time for becoming experienced in mucus and cervix observations and to establish a minimum of six cycles as a basis for cycle variation.

Once you have basis of six or more cycles, the 21-day rule can be used with great effectiveness to allow coitus in Phase I with a minimum of risk. Couples using this rule of thumb should draw a line on the chart at the beginning of the cycle to indicate the limits of Phase I under the 21-day rule. For example, if the shortest cycle had been 27 days, then day 6 would be the limit of Phase I with this rule of thumb, and a line should be drawn between the temperature-recording lines for days 6 and 7.

Pre-ovulation Base

During the learning stage and whenever a chart is to be submitted for counselling purposes, it is recommended that the couple draw a line showing the judgment of the pre-ovulation base. This is set primarily by the normal highs of the six temperatures before the post-ovulation rise in temperature begins.

Thermal Shift Level

As above, during the learning stage and whenever a chart is to be submitted for counseling purposes, it is recommended that the couple draw a line showing the level of the thermal shift. This will normally be 4/10 of a degree above the pre-ovulation base.

Notation of the Beginning of Phase III

With many charts, the coitus notation makes it apparent when the couple judged Phase III to begin. However, for various reasons many couples will not have coitus on the very first day of the absolutely infertile period. For counseling and educational purposes, it is necessary for the counselor to know how the couple themselves have interpreted the chart. Therefore, we ask couples to draw a line on the chart indicating the beginning of Phase III.

70

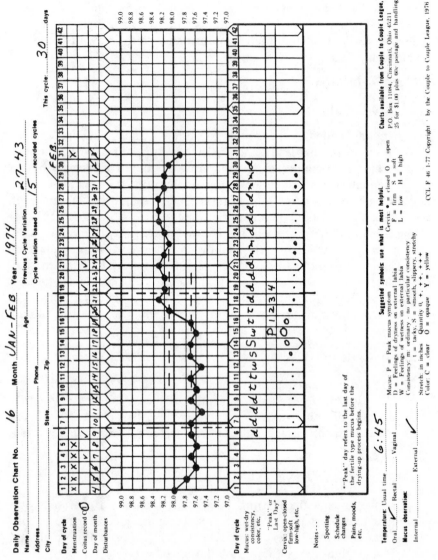

Figure 5.2: A Well Completed Chart

The chart Fig. 5.2 illustrates most of the notations to be made. The *Coitus record* line is incomplete; thus the "I" is circled. The dotted line between days 6 and 7 indicates that day 6 is considered the last safe day according to the 21-day rule. The pre-ovulation temperature base is established at 97.7°. The thermal shift level is 98.1°. The dotted line between days 18 and 19 indicates that day 19 is the beginning of Phase III according to all the signs of ovulation.

6

The Interpretation of Charts

Most of us learn best by example. This chapter provides many examples that illustrate different types of cycles and some of the variations in signs and symptoms of ovulation that are seen on some charts.

The chapter is entitled "The Interpretation of Charts," but let us keep clear what that means. The charts are only a visible record of the various signs that have been occurring in a woman's body. Thus, the interpretation of charts really means "the interpretation of signs of fertility."

Section A. Guidelines for Interpretation

In interpreting these signs or symptoms, certain rules or guidelines are followed. These are based on the following scientific facts, which have already been mentioned:

1. Cervical mucus appears several days prior to ovulation. It reaches a peak of clearness, stretchiness, and wetness about a day *before* ovulation.

2. Changes in the cervix itself take place both before and after ovulation.

3. *After* ovulation, the corpus luteum secretes progesterone, which does three things of interest to natural family planning.

   (a) It suppresses further ovulation.

   (b) It causes the basal body temperature to rise.

   (c) It increases the viscosity of cervical mucus (i.e., makes it less fluid).

4. After ovulation, a second ovulation may occur; however, it will occur only within 24 hours of the first ovulation (due to the action of the progesterone as mentioned above).

5. The ovum is capable of being fertilized for about 24 hours after ovulation. Our rules must allow for the lifespan of the ovum from a possible second ovulation.

6. Sperm are capable of fertilizing the ovum for about 3 days (72 hours)

after sexual relations under normal conditions of fertility, although there is both shorter and longer life under certain conditions. (For further explanation of these matters, see Chapters 3 and 4.)

The first set of guidelines deal with determining the limits of Phase I, the time of pre-ovulation relative infertility. Second, there is a brief reminder about Phase II. Third, there are guidelines for determining the start of Phase III, the time of post-ovulation absolute infertility.

I. Guidelines for the End of Phase I, the time of pre-ovulation infertility.

Throughout this manual it is stressed that pre-ovulation infertility is called the phase of *relative* infertility; we also call it Phase I of the fertility cycle. We call it "relatively" infertile because it will be followed by fertility and ovulation (while Phase III is infertile because it consists of days well past ovulation). Therefore it is important to determine the end of Phase I — or the beginning of Phase II — with a high degree of accuracy. Different guidelines have been developed. Some provide a higher effectiveness and more continence while another may provide a longer estimate of Phase I but with reduced effectiveness. In each case, the first day of menstruation is counted as day 1 of the cycle. However, a bloody discharge cannot be regarded as a true menstruation unless it has been preceded by a sustained thermal shift. (See the section on breakthrough bleeding in conjunction with Figure 6.7 later in this chapter.)

1. **Complete continence.** Total continence in Phase I is one option and obviously has the lowest surprise pregnancy rate. Starting continence on the first day of menstruation yields a surprise pregnancy rate of zero. Treating the days of heavy flow as still in Phase III and starting continence on the first day of light flow would yield a surprise pregnancy rate close to zero.

2. **Day 4 guideline.** CCL Central has observed only 1 recorded pregnancy resulting from coitus on cycle day 4. Although there are no scientifically controlled studies that can be quoted for an effectiveness rate, the extensive experience of the members of the CCL Medical Advisory Board suggests that coitus on day 4 yields a surprise pregnancy rate no greater than that for surgical sterilization.

3. **Day 5 guideline.** CCL Central has observed only one pregnancy resulting from coitus on cycle day 5. Again, no scientifically controlled study can be quoted, but the experience of the CCL Medical Advisory Board indicates that cycle day 5 is an extremely infertile day. Based on this experience and the study of Dr. Roetzer regarding day 6, it is estimated that coitus on day 5 would have a surprise pregnancy rate of no more than 1/2 of 1% (1 per 200 woman years) provided that 1) the

woman has not had previous cycles of 22 days or less, and 2) there is still no detectable mucus on day 5. Therefore, the great majority of couples are able to use a day 5 guideline even when first learning the sympto-thermal method.

4. **Day 6 guideline.** In the study reported by Dr. Josef Roetzer in 1968[1] couples used day 6 as the end of Phase I. The overall pregnancy rate from this study was 0.7 per 100 woman years. In personal communications Dr. Roetzer has mentioned the experience of one couple where the woman had a history of 22 day cycles. In this experience, coitus on day 5 did not result in pregnancy, but a pregnancy did occur as soon as they began to have coitus on day 6.

Based on his work and on the clinical experience of the other members of the CCL Medical Advisory Board, it is estimated that the pregnancy rate for coitus on day 6 is less than 1 per 100 woman years provided that 1) the woman has not had previous cycles of 22 days or less and 2) there is still no detectable mucus on day 6. Thus a big majority of couples will be able to use a day 6 guideline even when first learning the sympto-thermal method.

5. **Day 7 guideline.** Clinical experience has shown that fertility returns with increasing frequency starting with cycle day 7. Couples having coitus on day 7 or later should regard themselves in Phase I only on the basis of the following guidelines (the 21 day rule and the detection of mucus):

6. **The 21-Day Rule of Thumb.**
This guideline is based on previous cycle history and can be stated as follows:
"Shortest previous cycle minus 21 yields the last day of Phase I, provided that mucus is not present on or before that day."
Some examples of the 21 day rule follow:

Shortest Cycle	Minus 21	Last day of Phase I
32	-21	11
30	-21	9
28	-21	7
26	-21	5

It should be noted that the 21-day rule is *subordinate to the presence of early mucus* which provides a positive indication of the start of Phase II, the fertile time. Therefore, if the 21 day rule indicated day 8 as the end of Phase I but mucus was present on that day, the couple should regard themselves as already in Phase II.

One basis for the 21-day rule is that ovulation may occur from 10 to 16 days before the next menstruation, and sperm under some conditions may live up to 5 days. The rule is conservative and uses the 16 and 5 day figures. By using these figures it also tends to make allowance for an ovulation that might occur one or two days earlier than in any previously recorded cycle. A practical basis for this guideline is that too many surprise pregnancies occurred when a 19 day guideline was used, so the rule of thumb was extended to 21 and has been working very well.

How do you know the shortest previous cycle? Here is seen the importance of accurate record keeping. A couple must have accurate cycle length records before the 21-day rule can be meaningful. The more records they have, the better. How many months' records are necessary? Dr. John Marshall has studied this extensively. On the basis of 4,593 cycles he concluded that at least six cycles should be known to make a fairly accurate prediction about future cycle lengths. In his study he found that with six months' records of cycle lengths, 82 percent of the next three cycles fell within the same range; if there were twelve months' records, 90 percent of the next three cycles fell within the already recorded range. However, on the basis of three months' records, only 64 percent of the next three cycles were within the range.[2]

This means that if Mrs. A has three months of cycles showing a range of 28 to 30 days, there is about one chance in three that at least one of her next three cycles will be either shorter or longer than the 28 to 30 day range. If she has a year's record showing that same range of 28-30 days, then the chance is only one in ten that one of her next three cycles will be shorter or longer than that range.

Thus CCL recommends that a couple should have at least six or more cycles of experience before applying the 21 day rule of thumb.

The 21-day guideline is not applicable when a woman has a luteal phase of more than 16 days. Thus, if a woman has more than 16 days of rising and elevated temperatures, the couple should add one day to the 21-day guideline for every extra day (beyond 16) of elevated temperatures to formulate their own rule of thumb. In all such cases, the wife should be very observant for appearance of mucus.

The 21-day rule of thumb may be modified for short cycles in accord with the guidelines for cycle days 4, 5 and 6 given above.

Based on wide clinical experience but without a scientifically controlled study, we estimate that the correct application of the 21 day rule will yield a surprise pregnancy rate of about 1% (1 per 100 woman years).

7. Detection of early mucus.

Without the presence of cervical mucus, sperm life is very short and is measured in terms of a few hours rather than days. The appearance of early mucus provides a positive sign of the start of Phase II, the fertile time. Thus, before the beginning of the mucus symptom, "dry days" may be used for coitus with a high probability of natural infertility. Such a practice can extend Phase I beyond the limits of the previous guidelines, especially in longer cycles, thus requiring less continence than may be required by the other rules of thumb.

Since the effectiveness of this guideline depends upon the woman's ability to detect such mucus when it starts, certain precautions should be followed.

A. The Experience Factor:

Do not rely upon the detection-of-early-mucus guideline until the woman has had at least six cycles of experience and has developed both ability and confidence in the detection of the mucus sign.

B. Alternate-dry-days-only rule:

1. Do not have coitus on consecutive days in Phase I, especially after cycle day 6. (The woman might misinterpret mucus discharge as being only the seminal residue from the night before.)

2. Do not have coitus on days on which cervical mucus is present.

C. Other Important Considerations:

1. *How effective is the alternate-dry-days-only rule?*

In theory, it is highly effective. In practice, some women may have difficulties detecting the beginning of mucus, and thus may have coitus in the beginning of Phase II. It would seem safer to follow the alternate-dry-days-only rule in cases where the woman consistently has a relatively long period of mucus preceding ovulation than in cases where mucus is observed for only two to five days before it starts to dry up and disappear.

Based on several studies by others, [3,4,5] CCL estimates that the alternate-dry-days-only rule provides a surprise pregnancy rate between 3 and 7% (3 to 7 pregnancies per 100 woman years).

Since these studies were based on mucus detection only by the sensation of wetness on the lips of the vulva and observations of toilet tissue, the effectivenss may possibly be improved through the Keefe method of mucus detection. This consists of inserting two fingers into the vaginal tract, gently but firmly "milking" the cervix, keeping the fingers together as they are withdrawn, and then examining for stretchability and the other signs of fertile-type mucus. Such a method may detect mucus a day before it is noticeable on the outer lips of the vulva or in the vagina.

2. *Are the days of menstruation infertile?*

The day or days of heavy flow may be regarded as an extension of Phase III of the last cycle and thus "absolutely infertile."

The days of the light or waning flow through day 5 as described above may be considered as still in Phase I (but see also the next question).

If a flow extends beyond day 5, the couple should postpone coitus until the establishment of post-menstruation dry days so that the menstrual flow would not mask the observation of an early mucus discharge.

3. What if mucus appears on day 4, 5 or 6 or before the end of Phase I as defined by the 21 day rule?

Such days must be regarded as possibly fertile, and coitus should be avoided by those seeking to postpone pregnancy. However, as a matter of fact, the appearance of mucus and fertility on days 4, 5 or 6 is an extremely rare event as previously indicated.

4. Is coitus "relatively infertile" on the days after menstruation and before ovulation when early mucus may be merely tacky, that is, when it does not yet have the lubricative, clear and stretchy characteristics of the most fertile type of mucus?

Some advocates of the mucus-only method have called this pre-ovulation, tacky, opaque mucus "infertile-type mucus" and have said that experienced couples who could really tell the difference in mucus types could regard such days as being relatively infertile. However, a number of pregnancies have been observed from coitus on such days. Thus, the general rule must be to regard pre-ovulation days of tacky mucus as indicating fertility.

5. During very long cycles sometimes mucus appears and disappears. Are any days in this pattern relatively infertile?

If mucus is only of the "less-fertile type" described above, then the dry days should be relatively infertile. However, if any mucus is of the clear and stretchy variety and/or produces the feeling of vaginal wetness or lubrication, such mucus is definitely of the more fertile type, and it must be assumed that ovulation is occurring, even if there is only one day of such mucus. The rule of "Peak + 4" must be followed. If such mucus is followed by four dry days, the fourth day may be regarded either as relatively or absolutely infertile. (If it was accompanied by a thermal shift, the absolutely infertile phase has begun. If there was no temperature rise, the woman is still in an extended Phase I according to the mucus sign.)

6. During Phase I, does it make any difference whether a couple has coitus in the evening or the morning?

Yes. A dry day is known only by the sum of the observations made during the day. However, the mucus may begin to flow during the night but still be undetected upon waking. Thus there is a greater probability of having an adequate mucus warning of fertility by **avoiding coitus in the morning** during Phase I.

7. Should couples follow the alternate-dry-days-only guideline if also following the 21 day rule or the guidelines for cycle days 4, 5 and 6?

It is advisable. It is possible at any time that a woman may mistake early mucus for seminal residue. Therefore, greater accuracy in early mucus detection will be gained by not having coitus on consecutive days at any time during Phase I.

8. *If a woman thinks that a vaginal discharge is simply seminal residue, should she continue to make periodic mucus observations that day?*

Very definitely yes. The mucus flow may also be beginning and the regular observations should be made and recorded.

II. Guidelines for the presence of Phase II, the fertile time.

In this text, the limits of Phase II, the fertile time, are described chiefly in terms of the end of Phase I and the beginning of Phase III. If, for example, the 21 day rule yielded day 7 as the end of Phase I, couples would regard Phase II as starting on day 8. The start of the mucus sign, as contrasted with the other Phase I guidelines, actually provides a positive sign of the start of Phase II. If mucus appears for the first time on day 8, the couple should regard themselves in Phase II.

The guidelines for Phase III describe the time of postovulation infertility as beginning on the evening of the day indicated by a particular guideline. Thus Phase II, the fertile time, is considered to continue until that time.

However, couples seeking to achieve pregnancy need to have a way of locating not just overall outer limits of the fertile time but also the time of greatest fertility. Aids for this are provided in conjunction with Figure 6.2 later in this chapter.

III. Guidelines for the Start of Phase III, the time of postovulation infertility.

Based on the biological facts and on practical experience, several guidelines have been developed to be used in different situations. In each case, Phase III, the time of postovulation infertility, begins on the evening of the day indicated. The term "full thermal shift" as used in these guidelines refers to the occurrence of at least three elevated temperatures that are *consecutively* at least 4/10 of one degree Farenheit above the pre-ovulation base. (See fuller description of the pre-ovulation base following the guidelines for Phase III).

A. *Four Basic Rules of Thumb*

1. **Perfect coinciding** (PC): The three primary signs coincide as follows to indicate the start of Phase III:
   a. The third day of full thermal shift.
   b. The fourth day of drying up or disappearance of mucus.
   c. The fourth day of the cervix closing or lowering.

PC can also refer to this crosschecking combination of mucus and temperature when usable cervix observations have not been recorded.

2. Rule C or FC (Final Coinciding): Frequently the mucus and temperature signs do not perfectly coincide. Rule C refers to the cautious and conservative interpretation that Phase III begins only when there are both (a) at least four (or more) days of mucus drying up *and* (b) three (or more) days of *full* thermal shift temperatures.

3. Rule A (more emphasis on temperatures): Phase III begins when a full thermal shift of three or more consecutive days has been corroborated (cross-checked) by at least two days of drying up or disappearance of the mucus.

Rule A can be used where the temperatures form a very sharp and unmistakable full thermal shift while the mucus sign is slower to indicate infertility. Wide clinical experience with temperature-only interpretations leads us to think that little is to be gained by waiting for more than 2 days of mucus drying up in the face of such a strong and clearly defined thermal shift. However, when the pre-ovulation base has been shaved or averaged, it is recommended to wait for 3 days of mucus drying up. (See the following Section IV, Additional Aids for the Interpretation of Temperatures.)

4. Rule B (more emphasis on mucus): Phase III begins when four or more days of drying up or dryness have been corroborated by the temperatures sign as follows: (a) there are at least three days of temperatures above the pre-ovulation base; (b) these temperatures are in a rising and/or elevated pattern; (c) at least one or more of these temperatures has reached the normal thermal shift level of 4/10 of a degree above the pre-ovulation base.

Rule B assumes that the woman is well experienced in mucus observation.

Rule B can be used where the mucus sign is very clear in its indication of infertility while the temperature rise is slower to form a full thermal shift. In such cases, the type of rising or elevated temperature pattern described in Rule B is satisfactory to provide crosschecking for the mucus symptom. Thus, the Rule B interpretation accepts an overall rising or elevated temperature pattern which does not meet the stricter requirements of a "full thermal shift" described above.

When the signs do not coincide, the more conservative approach is to use the Rule C guideline. However, our own experience and the published research of others leads us to believe that the proper application of Rules A and B by experienced couples produces excellent results with a surprise pregnancy rate of only about one per cent (one per 100 woman years of exposure).

B. *More Guidelines for Special Situations*

1. **Just starting.** Beginners should add at least one day to all rules of thumb as a precaution against their own possible misinterpretation of the signs. This would also hold true in cases where only one sign was being used without corroboration from the other signs, a practice not really recommended by the Couple to Couple League.

2. **Utmost need to avoid pregnancy.** When the signs do not coincide perfectly, couples having the most serious need to avoid pregnancy are advised to follow the Rule C interpretation of waiting for both four (or more) days of mucus drying up *and* three (or more) days of full thermal shift. They may also want to follow the beginner's guideline of always adding an additional day as an extra precaution. Based on the Vincent[6] temperature-only study, we estimate that the Rule C interpretation should yield a surprise pregnancy rate no greater than those for sterilization, and that the policy of Rule C plus one day should be even *more* effective.

3. **Just-off-the-Pill.** Women coming off the oral contraceptive Pill may have a confusing mucus pattern in the first few cycles off the Pill. In the presence of a very clear and sustained full thermal shift, it is not necessary to wait for corroboration from the mucus: it may never come in that cycle. Thus the following temperature-only guideline has been developed for assistance in cycles just off the Pill.

"Phase III begins on the evening of the fifth day of an elevated or rising temperature pattern in which at least the last three temps are consecutively at the full thermal shift level."

This interpretation assumes the absence of the more fertile type of mucus. It can be used despite the presence of all-the-time-merely-tacky mucus due to hormonal residues.

4. **Temperature-only.** Sometimes a woman finds no indications of fertility or infertility from the mucus or cervix signs. This means that she is unable to recognize mucus or has a continuous discharge of tacky mucus which prevents recognition of any changes. Yet she experiences a thermal shift. For such cases, the following guideline has been developed:

"Phase III begins in the evening of the fourth day of a rising or elevated temperature pattern in which at least the last three have been at the full thermal shift level." This guideline envisions either a full thermal shift of 4 days or a 4 day pattern starting with a day of partial rise and concluding with a 3 day full thermal shift.

5. **Note on cervix.** Some experienced women may find cervix signs very usable even in the absence of usable mucus signs and thus use the cervix signs as an adequate substitute for the mucus signs in the above rules of thumb for both the beginning and the end of phase II.

IV. Additional Aids for the Interpretation of Temperatures

The Pre-ovulation base

Experience has shown that the most difficult part of temperature interpretation is the determination of the pre-ovulation base. The following comments are intended to review and clarify the situation.

Definition: The pre-ovulation base is the level from which the post-ovulation rise is measured.

The pre-ovulation base (POB) is determined by the normal highs among the six temperatures just before the overall postovulation rise which makes up the thermal shift. It should be noted that to establish the pre-ovulation temperature base, it is necessary to have at least six days of temperature records before the beginning of the postovulation rise. Sometimes experienced couples reduce the number of temperature recordings too much and are left with an insufficient number of recordings to determine a meaningful pre-ovulation base (see fig. 6.15, for such an example.) The normal amount of difference between the POB and the thermal shift level is 4/10 of 1° F.

The six temperatures used to determine the pre-ovulation base are called the pre-shift six.

Some examples of setting the pre-ovulation base:

Turn back to Figure 5.2. In that chart, the POB is easily established at 97.7 and the thermal shift level (TSL) is at 98.1.

Now turn ahead to Figure 6.1. The POB is set at 97.8. The temperature on day 14 is slightly above the previous six but not at the full thermal shift level. This is a day of mini-rise and is not counted among the pre-shift six. (It could be counted as the first mini-shift temperature in applying the 4-day temperature-only guideline.)

The occasional difficulty in establishing the POB is illustrated in this example:

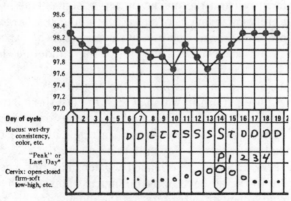

EXAMPLE 1. SHAVED POB: 97.9° F.

By day 18 it is apparent that a definite shift in levels has occurred and has been accompanied by a mucus dry-up pattern. However, the application of the CCL standard guidelines is hindered by the irregular high on day 11. If we used day 11 to establish the POB at 98.1, the normal thermal shift requirement of 4/10 of 1° F. is not met.

A well experienced couple or NFP counselor would simply ignore the temperature on day 11 on the basis of experience with overall patterns, but less experienced couples want and need some rules to follow. The CCL approach to this situation has been the development of the following guidelines:

1. Shaving the highs.

General principle: When the interpretation of an otherwise obvious shift in temperature levels is held up by one or two higher temperatures among the pre-shift six, these higher temps may be shaved slightly in order to get a standard application of the basic guidelines (a "guidelines fit").

a. The first step is to shave down the one or two temperatures by 1/10 of 1° F.

b. If that does not produce a guidelines fit, shave down the one or two irregular highs to the next highest level among the rest of the pre-shift six. In Example 1 above, the temperature on day 11 was shaved down to the level of the next highest temperatures in the pre-shift six, and the POB was thus established at 97.9°.

c. In some cases, the pre-ovulation base may be determined by the arithmetic average of the pre-shift six. However, the practice of averaging is quite open to misinterpretation and is therefore not recommended, especially for inexperienced couples. It can lead to cutting corners, disregarding the other signs of ovulation in the face of a very slight sustained temperature rise, and erroneous estimation of the pre-ovulation base level. In addition, a true "average" would involve both addition and division and introduce usually unnecessary calculations into the process.

Shaving the highs or averaging should be done only —
1. if it is truly necessary to produce a guidelines fit,
2. if there is an otherwise visually obvious thermal shift,
3. if the shift is accompanied by three or more days of mucus drying up.

In the vast majority of cases, the highest temperature reading or readings among the last six pre-shift temperatures are the ones that truly set the pre-ovulation base. On the other hand, in some cases it is helpful to do some "shaving" or "averaging" in conjunction with the other signs of ovulation.

False Rises and Unexplained Temperature Elevations

Throughout this manual, the postovulation thermal shift is described as a sustained temperature elevation at least 4/10 of a degree above the pre-ovulation base, and occurring as the cervical mucus sign disappears. However, pre-ovulation temperatures may occur that are above the general level of the rest of the temperatures, and a decision must be made whether to determine the pre-ovulation base level by the higher temperature, to exclude it, or to shave it as mentioned previously.

The following guidelines should be used to arrive at such a decision:

1. High temperature readings that are obviously due to a fever or some lesser illness such as a bad cold or a sore throat should be disregarded.

2. The alcohol from a couple of drinks the night before can influence the next morning's basal temperature.

3. Arising later than usual typically yields a higher temperature. A change in daylight saving time has the effect for about 2 or 3 days of rising an hour earlier (slightly lower temperatures) in the spring and rising an hour later (slightly higher temperatures) in the fall.

4. An unaccustomed chill or heat may affect the basal temperature. For example, one woman had an apparent three-day thermal shift but she was sure that ovulation had not occurred due to the absence of the pre-ovulation signs. This mother, who always slept with her baby, remembered that on each of those three mornings her five-year-old had crawled into her bed several hours prior to the temperature-taking time. She reasoned the second child's close presence must have given additional warmth to her body.

These are all explainable causes due to erratic temperature elevations and are sometimes called "false rises"; examples that discount these types of false rises are provided in some of the charts in this chapter.

However, in some cycles, one or two temperature readings may occur that cannot be explained by the above types of causes. Sometimes, such unexplained rises may be of no concern, but at other times the couple may wonder if the pre-ovulation base level should be affected by them. Inexperienced couples should seek help from an experienced Couple to Couple League counselor, who would consider the following factors:

1. Does the questioned temperature reading make any difference, or has the postovulation temperature risen to at least 4/10 of a degree even above it?

2. If the pre-ovulation base is set without the questionable temperature, is a thermal shift from *that* level corroborated by the mucus and/or cervix signs of ovulation? If so, the questionable temperature may be shaved.

3. When in the pre-shift phase of the cycle did the questionable temperature elevation occur? If it was seven or more days before the thermal shift, it can be ignored.

4. How many "questionable" temperatures are there? One and sometimes two temperatures may be unexplained "false rises" that can be shaved or discounted. Three or more are pattern setting, not erratic, and would have to be considered in establishing the pre-ovulation base, either as setting the pre-ovulation base by their highs or at least to be used in calculating an average.

Thermal Shifts of Less Than the Normal Amount

A few women regularly show a thermal shift pattern that is less than the normal shift of at least 4/10 of a degree. Well instructed couples can learn to interpret such rises *in conjunction with the other signs of ovulation* and successfully use the sympto-thermal method. A cross drawn on the chart in such a way that the horizontal line is *above* six temperatures to the left of the vertical line and *below* three (preferably four) temperatures to the right of the vertical line can help in determining the thermal shift in conjunction with the other signs of ovulation. Normally, the judgement on such a pattern should be discussed with experienced natural family planning counselors.[7]

Postovulation Dip

Sometimes there is a marked dip in the temperature readings after the thermal shift. If a dip to the pre-ovulation level occurs after the sustained thermal shift (as determined by the three-to-five-day counts mentioned in the various guidelines above), then it may be disregarded. However, in the temperature-only system, Marshall suggests that if such a dip occurs *before* the three-to-five-day counts of temperature rise indicate the beginning of the infertile phase, then the count must begin over again after the dip.[8]

In the sympto-thermal system, if a dip occurs while the thermal shift is apparently taking place, it can be treated under the Rule B guidelines if it has not dipped *to* or *below* the pre-ovulation base.

However, if the temperature has dipped to or below the pre-ovulation base, then the count should start over again. If a woman is well experienced in mucus and/or cervix signs and if these indicate post-ovulation infertility, and if the overall pattern prior to the dip was well elevated or rising, some couples may require for themselves only two temperatures — or even one — beyond the dip to confirm the pre-dip rising trend; but the general rule should be to require three rising or elevated temperatures beyond such a dip to corroborate the other signs and symptoms.

Irregular Temperature Patterns

The greatest aid to the interpretation of temperatures are the natural ovulation signs of mucus and cervix, and for most couples the following data on various temperature interpretations may thus be unnecessary. However, in cases where the woman is having difficulty in learning to observe or interpret the mucus and/or cervix signs, this information may be helpful. Our chief source for the rules of thumb with regard to the first three patterns — the slow rise, the step rise, and the zigzag rise — has been Marshall.[9]

The Slow Rise

In some cycles (14 percent according to Marshall[10]) a slow rise in temperatures occurs that usually reaches the anticipated thermal shift of 4/10 of a degree over several days (see example 2).

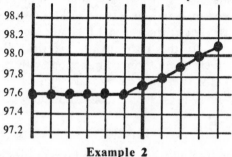

Example 2

The following guideline may be helpful in such cases. Starting with the first temperature that is above the pre-ovulation base, count five days instead of the usual three.[11] This assumes that all the five temperatures are higher each day. If the temperatures dip to or below the pre-ovulation base, however, the count must start over again. At least the last temperature must have reached an elevation of 4/10 of a degree above the pre-ovulation base.

The Step Rise

A small percentage of charts (3 percent according to Marshall[12]) show a steplike upward progression (see example 3).

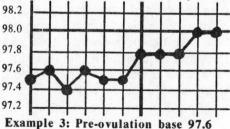

Example 3: Pre-ovulation base 97.6

The rule of thumb is the same as for the slow rise. Beginning with the first temperature above the pre-ovulation base, count five days of ascending temperatures and consider the fifth day as the beginning of an infertile phase. Again, at least the last temperature must have reached the level of 4/10 a degree above the pre-ovulation base.

The Zigzag Rise

Somewhat similar to the step-rise charts are those patterns that move upward in a zigzag fashion (see example 4).

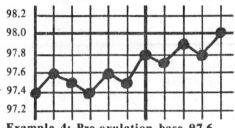

Example 4: Pre-ovulation base 97.6

Provided that the dips do not go to or below the pre-ovulation base, the rule of thumb is the same for the step rise, and at least the last temperature must have reached the level of 4/10 of a degree above the pre-ovulation base.

With regard to all three of these guidelines, Marshall[13] offers the caution that in cases of the most serious need to avoid pregnancy, couples should require three days of temperatures at the normal full thermal shift level of 4/10 of 1° F. above the pre-ovulation base. Thus, although we recognize that in most cases a five day rising temperature pattern in the absence of discernible mucus and cervix signs of fertility provides a good indication of being in Phase III, we prefer to use these temperature patterns in conjunction with Rule B interpretations. Thus we prefer to recommend the use of the four-day-temperature-only guideline in cases where no help is provided by the mucus and cervix symptoms.

(The very nature of CCL as a teaching organization calls for conservative recommendations, and couples with lesser need to avoid pregnancy can modify our preferred recommendations accordingly.)

Agreement or Nonagreement Among the Signs

What if mucus, cervix, and temperature signs do not all seem to agree? In figure 6.1, all three of these signs coincide perfectly. However, at times there will not be such a perfect relationship. In cases where there is an apparent conflict between mucus and basal temperature, precedence normally should be given to the temperature indications; — thus Rule B interpretations require a minimum of 3 days of temperature corroboration. The reasons for generally giving precedence to the basal temperature guidelines are as follows:

1. There has been more scientific documentation of the reliability of the basal temperature rules. When couples postpone coitus until the third day of a true thermal shift, surprise pregnancies are extremely rare — almost unknown.

2. Some women are less adept at recognizing mucus signs than they are at making accurate temperature recordings, particularly if they are inexperienced. The same holds true with the cervix.

3. If the temperature rise is delayed for several days beyond when it would normally be expected according to the mucus sign, we do not *know* why; however, we theorize that one cause may be a delayed production of progesterone, which is responsible for the natural suppression of further ovulation in that cycle. It is, in fact, not unusual for the temperature to begin rising not on the day after ovulation, but on the second or even third day after ovulation.

4. Thus, while CCL provides a temperature-only guideline, it does not provide mucus-only or cervix-only guidelines. If couples decide to establish such guidelines for themselves, we offer the caution that they should not regard themselves in Phase III until the temperature sign has given its corroboration. Thus if a couple believes they are infertile because the mucus has dried up for more than four days and the cervix has been closed for more than four days, they may consider themselves at best in a Phase I infertility and should apply the alternate-dry-days-only guideline. They should keep an accurate watch for the resumption of any mucus and cervix signs of fertility and regard themselves in Phase II if they re-appear.

Notes

Notes

Section B. Some Typical Examples

The interpretations of the following charts sometimes refer to specific rules of thumb. These are explained in the preceding section A.

A Normal Cycle

Fig. 6.1 shows the chart of a standard normal cycle. It illustrates several things.

In this example, the mucus sign makes its first appearance on day 8 and reaches peak mucus fertility on day 13. On days 14 and 15 it tapers off and has disappeared by day 16. "Peak of Mucus + 4" points to day 17 as the beginning of the absolutely infertile phase. Sometimes a slight amount of mucus appears in the postovulation infertile phase as on days 25-28. Since the temperature pattern has indicated the beginning of Phase III, such mucus is of no concern.

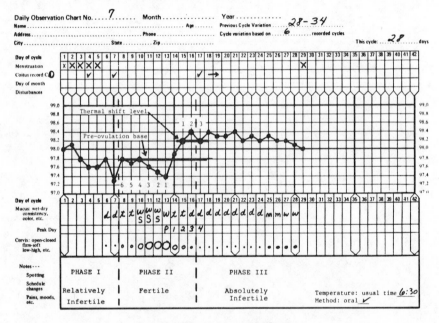

Figure 6.1 A Normal Cycle

Note that day 13—and not day 12—is the day of peak fertility according to the mucus sign. The symbols indicated that on day 13 the woman no longer noticed that the mucus was stretchy, but she still had a distinct feeling of wetness. On day 14 the feeling of wetness was gone and the mucus was merely tacky. Thus, day 14 is the first day of the drying-up process, and day 13 is called the day of the peak mucus symptom, the last day of the more fertile type mucus.

The cervix sign coincides with that of the mucus. The cervix begins to open slightly on day 8, reaches its largest opening on days 12 and 13, and begins to close again on day 14. "Closing day + 3" points to day 17 as the beginning of the infertile phase.

In analyzing the temperature graph, we are looking for a shift of temperature readings to a level that is at least 4/10 of a degree higher than the high level of the pre-ovulation temperatures. In fig. 6.1, among the six temperatures (for days 8-13) before the beginning of the post-ovulation rise, there are none higher than 97.8°, thus establishing the preovulation base at 97.8°. The normal thermal shift of at least 4/10 of a degree would yield basal temperature readings of 98.2° or more. In this example, this level begins on day 15. The third day of continued elevated basal temperatures is day 17, which thus becomes the first day of the absolutely infertile phase. Thus, all three signs coincide to indicate day 17 as the beginning of Phase III.

Note that day 14 is not counted as one of the three days of the thermal shift because it is only 1/10 of a degree above the 97.8° pre-ovulation base; nor is it counted in establishing the pre-ovulation base, because it is the first part of an overall rising pattern after ovulation.

Some temperature graphs show a basal temperature dip which is thought to occur just prior to or about the time of ovulation. It is seen in less than half of recorded cycles. It is of little significance to those desiring to avoid pregnancy, for two reasons. First, temperature dips may be due to other causes. In this example, there is a marked dip on day 7. Secondly, experience has shown that some couples who give attention to the dip have erroneously counted the temperature elevation as beginning from the bottom of the dip. Such a mistake can result in pregnancy. To repeat what has already been emphasized: To determine the beginning of the infertile phase by the basal temperature technique, look for a succession of at least three temperature recordings that are at least 4/10 of a degree higher than the *high level of the pre-shift temperatures.* (As a secondary aid to the interpretation of the charts, the dip can be helpful when mucus is present. It is a common opinion that when the two are present together, the dip indicates the approximate time of ovulation.)

The cycle range of 28-34 days based on 6 cycles would allow the application of the 21-day rule; both the 21-day rule and the appearance of mucus on day 8 would indicate day 7 as the last day of Phase I.

The *Coitus record* is noted as being an incomplete record. It indicates coitus within the limits of the 21-day rule, a 9-day period of continence, and the resumption of coitus on day 17, the first day of Phase III.

Trying to Become Pregnant

This chart (fig. 6.2) is inserted at the beginning of this chapter for two reasons. First, its presence here serves to emphasize that the Couple to Couple League is interested in assisting couples to understand the natural signs of fertility to achieve a pregnancy as well as to avoid it. Secondly, experience has shown that the majority of couples using CCL services desire to postpone or avoid a pregnancy, and the remainder of the charts are discussed from that point of view.

Couples who are unable to achieve a pregnancy are said to have a fertility problem. This may be due to one or more male factors such as insufficient sperm or to female factors such as insufficient mucus, excess acidity in the vaginal tract, blocked Fallopian tubes, or failure to ovulate. Some conditions may be corrected by a physician; some cases cannot be corrected and the couple must adjust to the fact that a pregnancy is not possible.

The Couple to Couple League is opposed to any form of artificial insemination, masturbation for seminal analysis, attempted "test tube" conception, and other forms of technological reproductive efforts on the grounds that these depersonalize the sexual act, which is meant to be a sacred act, an interpersonal renewal or affirmation of the couple's marriage covenant.

Perhaps as high as 80 percent of infertile couples have no apparent impediment to achieving a pregnancy and yet do not. Many of these cases may be due to something psychological, perhaps stemming from a superdesire to achieve a pregnancy. Such thinking derives from the observation that some couples, after long periods of trying, achieve pregnancy during adoption proceedings. There is little we can say to such couples except "relax," but others may be helped by the following comments about the timing of intercourse to maximize the possibility of conception.

The opening of the cervical os and the presence of cervical mucus indicate the approach of maximum fertility. Couples with a fertility problem should refrain from sexual relations for about five days before they try to achieve pregnancy in order to build up a maximum supply of sperm. This means that they will be looking for the time of greatest fertility for their first intercourse after this wait. Indicators that ovulation may be very close at hand include the following:

1. a temperature dip toward the end of the mucus pattern (sometimes indicates the day of ovulation);
2. the first drying-up day (frequently the day of ovulation);
3. the first day of temperature rise (may be within a few hours of ovulation).

In the case in fig. 6.2, the couple waited until day 15, the first day up from an apparent dip in temperatures. Day 18 was the second day of a feeling of wetness, and the cervix was more open than the day before.

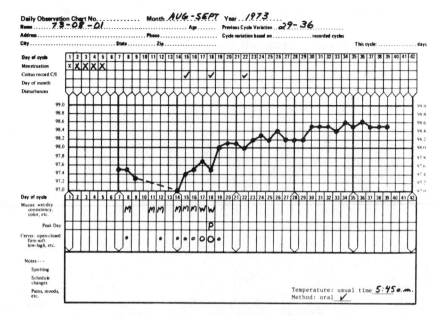

Figure 6.2 Achieving Pregnancy

It is impossible to say which instance of coitus was the one which led to this very-much-desired pregnancy, but from the indications provided, we would judge days 18 and 19 to be the most fertile days in the cycle. Any time from day 8 to day 21 would have to be considered fertile by a couple of normal fertility and ease of conception.

The pregnancy in fig. 6.2 was achieved about six months after attendance at CCL classes, indicating that even with proper understanding about maximum fertility and optimum timing, it still may take some time for everything to work together to provide the desired pregnancy.

If pregnancy is not achieved in the first month or two by timing coitus according to the ongoing signs of fertility, then a more systematic approach should be used. The couple desiring a pregnancy should carefully chart the signs and symptoms of ovulation and the daily basal body temperature for three cycles. The range of appearance and disappearance of mucus and the thermal rise should be observed. Days for coitus in the fourth cycle must be plotted in advance based on the days of maximum fertility of the three cycles already experienced. If in those three cycles the day of ovulation appeared to be days 13, 17, and 18 respectively, coitus in the fourth cycle should occur on days 14, 16, and 18. The first coital act should occur after a five-day period of abstinence to maximize the amount of sperm. The day of abstinence between coital acts allows sperm numbers to return to optimum level for fertilization, since daily coitus will deplete sperm and contribute to infertility.

The above system was used by fourteen couples attending Couple to Couple League meetings to seek assistance in achieving a pregnancy, and twelve of the couples achieved pregnancy within a few months.

An Earlier Ovulation in a Cycle of Normal Length

This chart (fig. 6.3) shows a slight variation from the previous one. Note the longer period of menstruation and that there were only three dry days before the beginning of mucus. The mucus phase was short and the phase between ovulation and the next menses was slightly longer than most. In both this and the preceding cycle, there were 16 days between the end of mucus and the beginning of the next menstruation. Ovulation probably occurred between days 10 and 13.

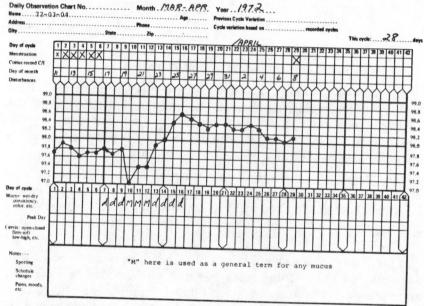

Figure 6.3 An Earlier Ovulation in a Cycle of Normal Length.

Two interpretations are possible in this case. Using the rule of three temperatures elevated 4/10 of a degree above the pre-ovulation high levels, only days 15, 16, and 17 can be counted. Day 17 is the beginning of the absolutely infertile phase.

A second interpretation would be possible *if we knew* that this woman was *experienced and accurate* in mucus observation. Since she did not note a peak, we would consider the last day of mucus as the peak, add four, and arrive at day 16. Does the temperature pattern corroborate this? The temperature of 97.9° on day 2 can be ignored because it occurred early in menstruation. The pre-ovulation base is thus 97.8°. Then, considering the slight temperature rise on days 13 and 14, which continued upward on days 15 and 16, it appears that the temperatures sufficiently backed up or corroborated the mucus signs to verify that day 16 is the first day of the absolutely infertile phase by Rule B.

A Relatively Short Cycle

The cycle illustrated in fig. 6.4 shows six days of menstruation followed immediately by five days of mucus. Since mucus may be difficult to observe during menstruation, it is possible that the mucus started even earlier.

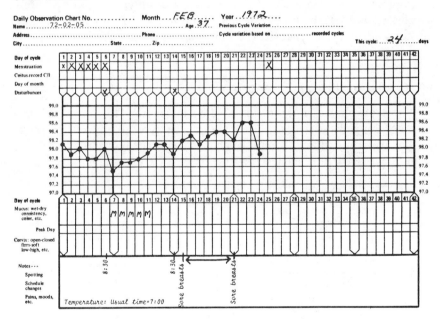

Figure 6.4 A Relatively Short Cycle

If at least six cycles showed none shorter than this 24-day cycle, application of the 21-day rule would yield day 3 as the end of Phase I. This could be modified to day 4 or 5 according to the Phase I guidelines given in Section A of this chapter. However, with a record of mucus starting on day 7 and the temperatures starting to rise on day 11, it would not be prudent to extend Phase I to day 6 in future cycles, especially if that was a day of menstruation.

94

The pre-ovulation base is 97.8 based on days 5-10 and shaving or discounting day 6 (late temp); the thermal shift level is 98.2.

The temperature and mucus signs do not coincide perfectly on this chart. Ordinarily this combination would yield a Rule B interpretation by day 15. However, the fact that the temperature dipped on day 14 in spite of being taken much later than usual raises a big question about what it might have been at the regular time. Thus we waited for two days of rising temps past the dip to confirm the trend set earlier by days 12 and 13. Thus Rule B yields day 16 as the start of Phase III.

The irregularity of the temperature taking during this cycle was not helpful. It forced a discounting or shaving on day 6, and it confused the reading on day 14. The mucus notations were very incomplete. The lack of notation after day 11 forced us to assume that dryness started on day 12, but such judgments should be based on definite, written notations. In this cycle there was a secondary symptom — sore breasts, a typical postovulation occurrence for this woman.

A Cycle of Longer Length

The cycle shown in fig. 6.5 is 33 days in length. This cycle, although slightly long, is still considered within the typical or average range.

The woman had been keeping records since her last child's birth and had records of four cycles ranging from 27 to 37 days.

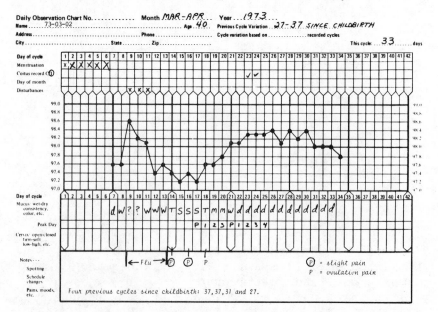

Figure 6.5 A Cycle of Longer Length

This chart shows why some women become pregnant using the old calendar rhythm. Because they ignored or had no record of the range of past cycles, they would plan on using the national statistical average. They would calculate safe and unsafe days on the basis of a 28-day cycle, estimate ovulation at the fourteenth day, and allow for three days on either side of ovulation for safety. Such a system is a mockery of the old calendar rhythm, but this is the kind of calculation that occurred in many cases. In this case, a "safety margin" of three days after the fourteenth day would set the first day of the absolutely infertile phase on day 18. On the contrary, it would be difficult to select a better day to conceive than day 18.

What about sexual intercourse during Phase I, the pre-ovulation, relatively infertile phase? The chart indicates only four menstrual periods since the last childbirth, and these were 37, 37, 31, and 27 days in duration. This couple chose not to have coitus during the relatively infertile phase. After at least six months of definite records, they would begin to apply the 21-day rule. If no cycles shorter than 27 days occurred, this would allow for coitus during the first six days of the cycle. In cases where the woman is positive of her mucus observations, some couples would also be relatively safe in having coitus on day 7 in a case such as this when it was a no-mucus or dry day.

In this case, the three high readings on days 9, 10, and 11 were due to the flu and are disregarded. The pre-ovulation base is 97.6°.

Peak mucus is indicated on day 17 and ovulation pain on day 18. However, on the day indicated by the rule of thumb "Peak Mucus + 4," day 21, a feeling of wetness is indicated, forcing the mucus count to begin over again, thus pointing to day 25 as the possible beginning of Phase III. Day 23 is the third day of a clear thermal shift. Since the signs do not coincide, Rule A may be applied to yield day 23 as the beginning of Phase III (third day of thermal shift corroborated by at least 2 days of drying up).

Long Cycles

The two charts in figs. 6.6a and 6.6b will be discussed together because they illustrate in different ways some of the same things about the sympto-thermal method.

The woman whose cycle is represented in fig. 6.6a normally had quite regular cycles; she was accustomed to begin her menstruation on day 28 or 29. However, this cycle was going to be much longer than usual for her. She experienced cramps on day 20 and a little mucus on days 20 and 21, but the temperature did not become elevated. By day 28 she convinced herself that she must have ovulated, that the temperatures were wrong. She fully expected menstruation to begin the next day and probably interpreted the cramps on days 28 and 29 as premenstrual. With this reasoning, the couple had coitus on day 28, apparently preferring to rely on past history rather than on the scientifically accurate data on her chart. As subsequent temperatures indicate, coitus occurred at the time of ovulation, and a pregnancy was the result.

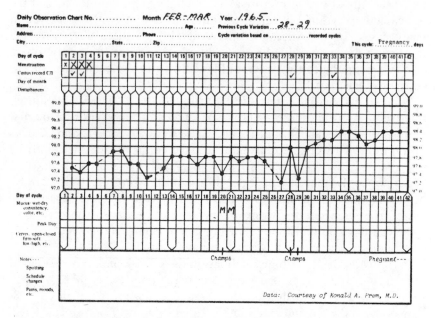

Figure 6.6a A Long Cycle and Lack of Confidence

This chart illustrates two important facts of life. First, the woman who normally is quite regular may experience an occasional cycle that is significantly different in length from the usual pattern. In this case, with ovulation at about day 28, this cycle would have been about 42 days long instead of her customary 28 or 29.

The sympto-thermal method with its ongoing observations is not upset by this change, whereas this marked variation made the old calendar rhythm (which was based only on past history) quite risky and likely to result in pregnancy. Secondly, this chart shows the importance of having confidence in the system of ongoing signs and observations. The scientific accuracy of these observations must continually be stressed by counselors.

The chart in fig. 6.6b was recorded by a woman whose cycles usually ranged between 35 and 40 days. This cycle was 59 days long. By the time she reached the limits of her usual cycle length, there was no sign of ovulation. Then on day 41 she began to experience some pain that she associated with ovulation, and on days 44, 45, and 46 she had definite mucus signs, with a peak of mucus on day 46. Day 48 was the first day of the thermal shift, and day 50 marked the third day of temperatures at a level at least 4/10 of a degree above the pre-ovulation base level of 97.9°. In arriving at the pre-ovulation base of 97.9°, we have discounted the higher readings that were apparently due to the temperature being taken at a later time or to other disturbances. Also, in determining the pre-ovulation base, the six temperatures immediately prior to the thermal shift should be given the most consideration.

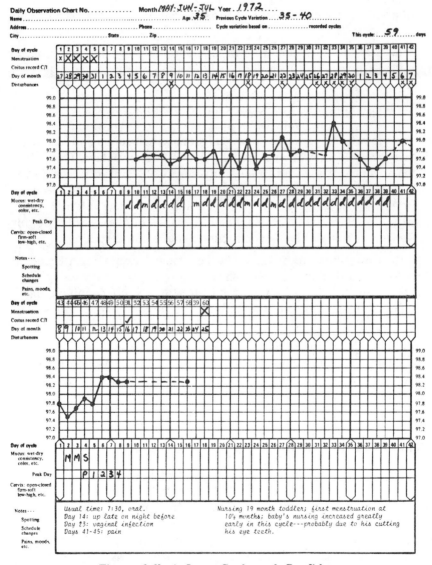

Figure 6.6b A Long Cycle and Confidence

The difference between the experience illustrated by the 59-day cycle in fig. 6.6b as contrasted with that in fig. 6.6a is that the couple with the 59-day cycle had confidence in the system. They had experienced previous pregnancies using the calendar rhythm system and had been using the sympto-thermal system for less than a year. The woman in this case commented that in previous years, if her menstruation had not occurred by the usual longest time (40 days in this case), they would have assumed that she was pregnant and would have begun having regular coitus. This chart indicated that ovulation had not occurred and the couple continued to wait.

Being strongly motivated to postpone another pregnancy, this couple refrained from coitus from very early in the cycle until day 51. This continence did no harm to their relationship.

Another couple who had less need to avoid pregnancy and who were willing to accept the small risk of pregnancy inherent in sexual relations during the relatively infertile phase might have had coitus on the mucus-dry days between days 9 and 39, but not on successive days. This is one of the advantages of accurate and daily mucus observations; however, it must be understood that sexual intercourse at any time during the cycle prior to the beginning of the postovulation, absolutely infertile phase carries a slight chance of pregnancy because of the possibilities of prolonged sperm survival or inaccurate mucus observations.

In the case illustrated by fig. 6.6b, the woman was not experienced in the cervix observation; however, she was able to note that on day 46 it was high while on day 47 it was low. Note also the perfect coinciding of the "Peak Mucus + 4" and the third day of elevated temperatures (day 50).

It should also be noted that the length of the cycle in this case was not entirely unexpected because of the great increase in breast-feeding early in the cycle. This is not at all unusual, and more will be said about it in Chapter 7.

Breakthrough Bleeding

In long cycles, bleeding may occur that begins like menstruation but really isn't. The endometrium builds up to such a degree that the very top layers cannot be sustained and are sloughed off. However, ovulation can occur at any time. The bleeding may be spotting or appear to be a regular period. If sexual relations occur during this period of bleeding, pregnancy can occur because the apparent menstruation is only break-through bleeding and ovulation may occur during it or immediately afterward. It is emphasized that this is a rare occurrence.

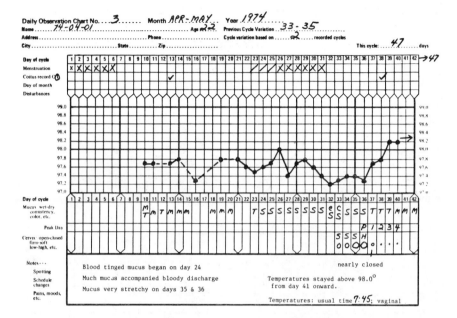

Figure 6.7 Breakthrough Bleeding

The chart in fig. 6.7 is a classic example of breakthrough bleeding occurring at the time of ovulation. The couple, who were in their third cycle of sympto-thermal observations, noticed that there were no indications of being in the absolutely infertile phase when they usually were in their previous cycles, about day 19. On day 24 the woman noticed the appearance of blood-tinged mucus and experienced over a week of mucus and bloody discharge, at the end of which she had clear and stretchy mucus before it began to dry up on day 37.

The pre-ovulation base is established at 97.4° by the six temperatures on days 31 to 36. All signs coincide to indicate day 40 as the beginning of Phase III. The cycle continued through day 47. The coitus on day 38 was too soon by any of the rules, but the couple were planning a pregnancy in a few months and decided gradually to cut down the days of continence.

It is important to realize that in this cycle there are two indications that the bleeding was not menstruation, which could be considered infertile. First of all, there was no thermal shift preceding it. It should be emphasized that a bloody discharge cannot be assumed to be menstruation unless it is preceded by a thermal shift, customarily about two weeks previously but sometimes shorter or longer. Secondly, the presence of mucus indicated possible fertility.

This chart illustrates the following rule for the interpretation of fertility during a bloody discharge. A bloody discharge may be considered to be menstrual bleeding and infertile only if:

1. It has been preceded by a thermal shift in the cycle that apparently has just ended.
2. It is within the limits of the 21-day rule.
3. No mucus is present.

Temperature Variations

This chart (fig. 6.8) illustrates two kinds of temperature variations that may appear on some temperature graphs.

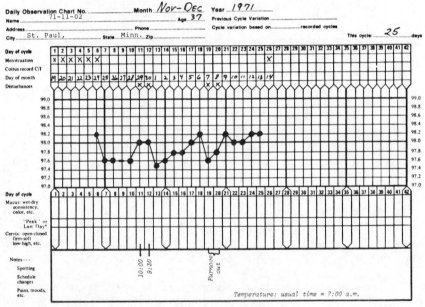

Figure 6.8 Temperature Variations

On days 11 and 12, the temperature was not taken until three hours and two and a half hours later than the usual time of 7 A.M. (Since such a practice is usually associated with sleeping later on Saturday and Sunday, it was surprising to check the calendar and find that November 29 and 30, 1971, were a Monday and a Tuesday.) The figure we have used earlier—a rise of 1/10 of a degree per half hour after the regular rising time—is only an average, but it would give us grounds to discount the temperatures on days 11 and 12 and regard them as probably no higher than 97.6° if they had been taken at the regular time. Such discounting is possible, but the recommended procedure is to take the temperature at the same time every day. If sleeping late, the woman should wake up long enough to take her temperature at the regular time and then go back to sleep. It can be extremely helpful if the husband sets the alarm at the usual temperature-taking time, gives the thermometer to his wife, and then puts the thermometer away five minutes later. Both may go back to sleep and record the temperature reading at a more convenient time during the day.

However, discounting days 11 and 12 leads us to accept 97.6° as the pre-ovulation base temperature level. A slight rise on days 15 and 16 is followed by temperatures on days 17 and 18 that are elevated 4/10 and 6/10 of a degree respectively.

Then, on day 19 a significant dip occurs, coincidental with the furnace having gone out during the night and the house having become thoroughly chilled. The furnace was not repaired until the next day, leaving two days' readings possibly affected by an overall chill in the house. The practical question: Should this couple decide that the dip on day 19 was due to the house chill and that the temperature reading would have been 98.2°, like the previous one, under normal conditions? Note that such an upward adjustment would make day 19 the third day of postovulation elevated temperatures and thus the first day of the postovulation infertile phase. (Note also that temperature variations due to external influence can occur in the opposite direction, giving false rises; for example, an overheated electric blanket.)

The answer must be "no" for the couple who do not wish to risk the possibility of a pregnancy. The general rule is that a dip to pre-ovulatory levels that occurs after one or two days of temperature elevations but before the third day cannot be disregarded, and counting must start again with the elevated temperatures after the dip, in this case with day 21. Thus, day 23 is considered the first day of the absolutely infertile phase.

However, if this woman had been experienced in making accurate observations of the mucus and cervical opening, it might have been a different story. In that case, if those signs had pointed to days 17, 18, or 19 as the beginning of the infertile phase, the dip could be ignored as being due to the chill, and the temperatures could be regarded as corroborating the other signs of ovulation. Thus, this chart illustrates the value of using the other signs of ovulation to assist in the interpretation of the temperatures.

102

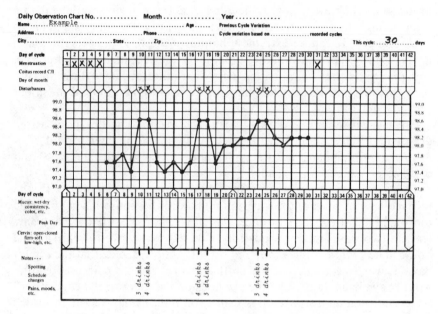

Figure 6.9 Alcohol and Temperature Variations

Alcohol and Temperature Variation

The chart in fig. 6.9 has been reconstructed from memory. A young engaged couple showed us a chart similar to this and gave us a copy, but unfortunately it was misplaced. What was striking about the chart at first glance was the very high temperature elevations occurring in doubles every seven days. Upon a closer look it became apparent that these were weekends, and, it turned out, this young couple liked to have a few drinks on their Friday and Saturday dates.

The purpose of including this chart is to illustrate that alcohol on the night before may have a very noticeable influence on the basal body temperature the next morning. In the light of this, it would seem quite practical to eliminate or greatly reduce any intake of alcohol during the time of ovulation and immediately afterward. "Discounting" never yields the same accuracy as basal temperature readings unaffected by alcohol, activity, later temperature-taking times, or other influences.

Many couples find it is more difficult to remain sexually continent when they have had a few drinks. Common sense should thus dictate a definite limitation on alcoholic intake during the times when the couple intend not to have sexual relations. In general, sobriety by both husband and wife will also spare many women the experience of participating in sexual intercourse that the wife knows has been initiated more by the influence of alcohol on her husband than by any real marital love and affection. Honest realization of this on the morning after does little to enhance a man's own self-respect.

Unexplained Temperature Elevations

Some women experience an unexplained rise in temperature about a day before the peak mucus sign and thus about two days before ovulation. The charts that have come to us are too inconclusive to say that this is a regular thing with these women; rather, our limited

104

observations lead us to see this as an irregular occurrence. We include mention of it because such a pre-ovulation rise can be somewhat confusing in establishing the pre-ovulation temperature base.

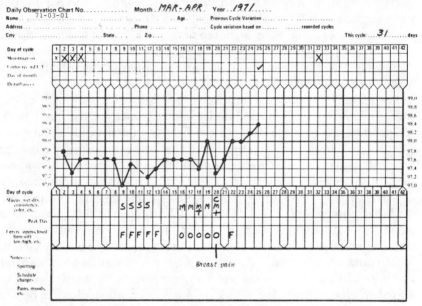

Figure 6.10a Pre-ovulation Temperature Elevation

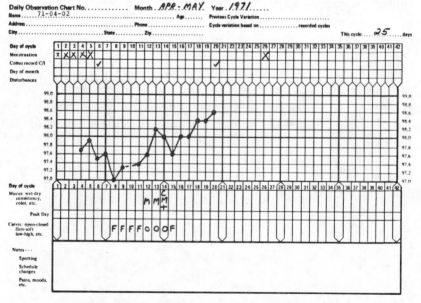

Figure 6.10b Pre-ovulation Temperature Elevation

For example, the charts in fig. 6.10a and 6.10b are from consecutive months from the same woman. The first chart has a pre-ovulation base of 97.6° until day 19, which is still before ovulation. By the time we reach day 22 we have to ask the question: Is the 98.0° reading of day 22 4/10 of a degree higher than the pre-ovulation base, or is it just equal with a pre-ovulation base regarded as 98.0° because of the reading on day 19?

In fig. 6.10b, the two slightly higher temperatures during the menstrual period should be disregarded. The pre-ovulation base then is 97.6° until the high readings of 98.2° and 98.0° on days 13 and 14, which are still before ovulation.

Because of this couple's rather long experience with basal temperatures and their ability to recognize and interpret the mucus and cervical signs of ovulation, they felt confident in disregarding the pre-ovulation "false rise" and accepted 97.6° as the pre-ovulation high level in both cases.

Thus, they were able to see day 24 in fig. 6.10a as the third day of temperatures elevated 4/10 of a degree or more above the pre-ovulation high level of 97.6°.

In doing so, they were helped greatly by the mucus sign, which peaked on day 20, and observation of the cervix, which was fully open on day 20 and firm on day 22. Similar things could be said about the chart in fig. 6.10b, where day 18 is the first day of the absolutely infertile phase.

Interestingly enough, in both charts the postovulation temperatures reached a point of 4/10 of a degree above even the "false rise" of the pre-ovulation phase. The couple apparently waited in these months until the temperature reached that point before they resumed coitus.

These examples illustrate that couples experienced in the sympto-thermal method of natural family planning need not be discouraged by some unexplained temperature elevations. By taking into consideration (1) the overall pre-shift level excluding the questionable temperature, (2) the mucus sign, (3) the cervix sign, and (4) the level of the postovulation thermal shift, the experienced couple can make intelligent decisions about "discounting" the questionable temperatures and can correctly determine the beginning of the absolutely infertile phase. The relatively inexperienced couple should seek help from counselors experienced in the art of interpreting charts.

106

Various Interpretations

The chart in fig. 6.11 illustrates several items: the need for a change in the cycle variation, a confusing mucus pattern, and an ambiguous temperature pattern. The previous cycle variation had been 31 to 37 days. This cycle was only 27 days long. Thus the cycle variation must be changed to indicate 27 to 37 days on the next chart. Application of the 21-day rule to that range in succeeding cycles would indicate day 6 as the end of Phase I.

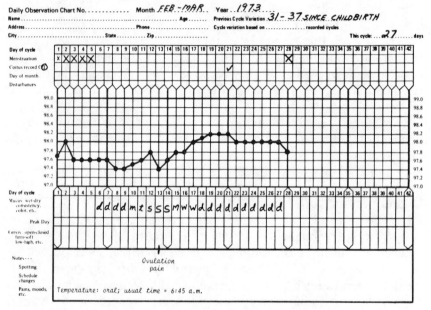

Figure 6.11 Various Interpretations

The woman had indicated day 14 as the day of peak mucus. In other words, she had noticed that the mucus was drying up on day 15, perhaps tacky and sticky, but at any rate no longer slippery or giving the feeling of wetness. However, on days 16 and 17 the feeling of wetness is again recorded, followed by dry days. Thus day 17 should have been labeled as the "peak" day, i.e., the last day before four days of dryness.

The temperature pattern is made ambiguous because of the 97.8° reading on day 12. It is the only such reading in the week before the temperatures gradually begin to rise on day 15.

Different interpretations are possible. The more conservative interpretation sets the pre-ovulation base at 97.8°. The thermal shift level is thus set at 98.2°, and the third day of thermal shift is day 21. This coincides perfectly with the fourth day of dryness, beginning the count of dry days with day 18.

A more liberal interpretation would average out the pre-ovulation base at 97.6°, thus setting the thermal shift level at 98.0°. Day 19 is the third day of thermal shift in this interpretation, corroborated by two days of drying up; it is also the fifth day of slow rise, which began with the 97.8° reading on day 15.

In such cases, the interpretation accepted by the couple will vary with their experience and need to avoid pregnancy. Inexperienced couples or those with a very serious need to avoid pregnancy would wait until all the signs had established the beginning of Phase III without any ambiguity (day 21 in this example). Those with much experience in their own temperature and mucus patterns and/or a lesser need to avoid pregnancy might choose the more liberal interpretation. The couple who handed in the chart chose the conservative course. The view from hindsight seems to confirm the liberal interpretation as permissible. That is, assuming 14 days between ovulation and the next menstruation and counting back from the beginning of the next menstrual period yields day 14 as the probable day of ovulation. However, couples have to make decisions based on the data at hand; hindsight is helpful only in the analysis of overall patterns.

Step Rise

The experienced woman who sent us this chart (fig. 6.12) noted that she thought it was a step rise with ovulation on the first rise. That meant that she thought that ovulation occurred on day 17.

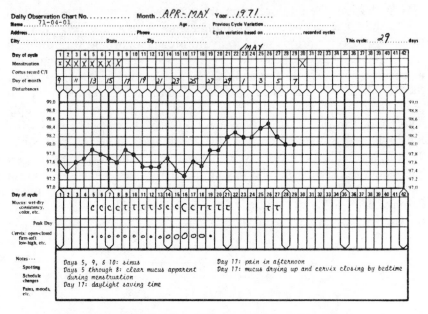

Figure 6.12 Step Rise Temperature Pattern

Looking at the signs of ovulation in the order in which this couple themselves experienced them, we see first of all the development of the mucus sign, "peaking" on day 17 with the drying-up process starting on day 18. This was paralleled by the opening of the cervix, which began closing on day 17. Thus, the cervix sign would point to day 20 as the first day of post ovulation infertility and the mucus sign would point to day 21. How well does the temperature corroborate either of these indications? The pre-ovulation base would be set at 97.7° (days 11-16). By day 20, two temperatures have been only 2/10 of a degree above the pre-ovulation base. Thus, the temperature on day 20 does not corroborate the cervix sign. On day 21, the temperatures have been above the pre-ovulation base for three days and have finally reached a level 4/10 of a degree above the pre-ovulation base. If the woman was experienced enough in the mucus observation to assure that the mucus was definitely drying up and almost gone, then the temperatures could be interpreted as confirming the mucus sign and indicating day 21 as the beginning of Phase III (Rule B).

Using the basal temperature guidelines only, both the 5-day step rise count begun on day 19 and the three days of elevated temperatures at the thermal shift of 4/10 of a degree would yield day 23 as the beginning of post ovulation infertility. Thus, in allowing day 21 as the first day of the infertile phase, the sympto-thermal interpretation here has obviously given heavy weight to the mucus and cervix signs, and this experienced woman looked only for a temperature rise that would corroborate, rather than independently confirm, the occurrence of ovulation.

Section C. Surprise Pregnancies and Learning from Others

It would be unfair to the readers of this manual to give the impression that there are no surprise pregnancies among couples who use natural family planning. As we noted previously, there is no such thing as a 100 percent method of conception regulation. At the same time, we noted that natural family planning can be as effective as any method (and more effective than most) if it is properly taught and learned, if there is sufficient motivation, and if it is practiced according to its rules. One study showed only one unplanned pregnancy in 17,500 cycles, a surprise pregnancy rate of about one per 1,458 woman-years of exposure.[14] Let us stress, however, that the couples in that study were well instructed and well motivated; they did not have coitus in the relatively infertile phase and waited until the temperature shift gave them clear indication of postovulation infertility; where the readings were ambiguous, they did not regard themselves in the absolutely infertile phase, and thus sometimes might not have had coitus during the entire cycle.

Most surprise pregnancies that occur in natural family planning are due either to lack of motivation or to misinterpretation by the couple.

The 1968 Marshall study[15] indicated that about 20 percent of the surprise pregnancies resulted from what the statisticians call a failure of the method. If the other 80 percent of surprise pregnancies resulted from the couples' lack of motivation or erroneous interpretation, then it may be profitable to look at some of these examples.

Surprise Pregnancies?

What is meant by a surprise pregnancy due to a lack of motivation? If a couple have been instructed that pre-ovulation mucus is associated with the time of highest fertility, and if the woman has noticed this mucus, and if they have coitus, can a pregnancy resulting from coitus at that time be called a "surprise pregnancy"? It seems to us that if this is a couple of normal fertility, the greater surprise would be if the woman did not become pregnant. Yet the rules for comparative statistics about birth control methods would have such a pregnancy counted as either a "method failure" or a "user failure." At any rate, the chart in fig. 6.13a illustrates such a case. We don't think of this case as any sort of "failure." Rather it simply illustrates that the presence of cervical mucus indicates fertility. The couple were not motivated to avoid pregnancy.

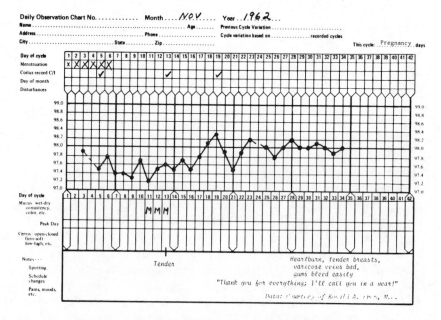

Figure 6.13a Lack of Motivation and Pregnancy

The chart in fig. 6.13b speaks for itself and illustrates another case where motivation was lacking. It certainly doesn't illustrate a "surprise pregnancy," but it does point to a difficulty and corresponding challenge of natural family planning. Yes, a little absence does tend to make the heart grow fonder. Yes, in a culture that tends to equate coitus with both "something to remember me by" and a "good way to say hello" there are additional subtle psychological inclinations toward coitus whenever a trip is begun or ended. But no, such coitus is by no means a necessity for a happy marriage. In such situations, the attitudinal stance of both partners, and perhaps the husband in particular, becomes very important. If every night that he has gone to bed alone in his hotel room (or at home if it is the wife who is traveling), he has looked forward to coitus upon their reunion, if perhaps the frequently sexually provocative costuming of airlines stewardesses has further turned his thoughts toward the marriage bed, and if this has not been pushed out of the imagination but rather been encouraged by a couple of drinks, then he is hardly engaging in the effort to grow in sexual maturity that is needed to practice natural family planning. Certainly the traveling man is usually going to want to embrace his spouse upon coming together again, but such an embrace need not include coitus. The sexually mature couple will be able to express the warmth, tenderness, and gentleness of marital love in a physical embrace without feeling a necessity to follow their erotic tendencies to their culmination in coitus. The next morning they may well have more satisfaction and self-esteem at having expressed their marital love in nongenital ways then if they had followed the cultural pattern of equating love-making with coitus.

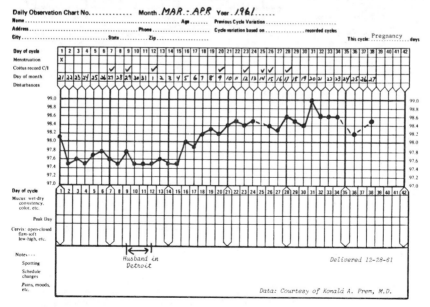

Figure 6.13b Absence, Lack of Motivation, and Pregnancy

112

The chart in fig. 6.13c shows coitus on day 20 prior to any sufficient indication of postovulation fertility. Note that this chart dates back to 1966, when no emphasis was given to the peak of mucus. Thus, we have no indication of any peak or of any changes in quality. This couple would, at that time, have been concerned almost completely with basal temperatures. With the pre-ovulation high level at 97.6°, the normally required 4/10 of a degree elevation would raise it to at least 98.0°. The day on which this couple had coitus, day 20, was only the first day of *any* rise above the pre-ovulation high level. Applying temperature-only theory to this chart, we would arrive at day 24 as the first day of postovulation infertility. If this woman was experienced in making mucus observations and had noted a peak on day 18 with dryness beginning on day 19 and continuing, we think that the pattern of temperatures by day 22 (but not sooner) would give sufficient corroboration to the mucus rule of "peak + 4" to regard day 22 as the first day of postovulation infertility. By either account, coitus on day 20 was either two or four days too soon. The rules were not followed, and pregnancy resulted.

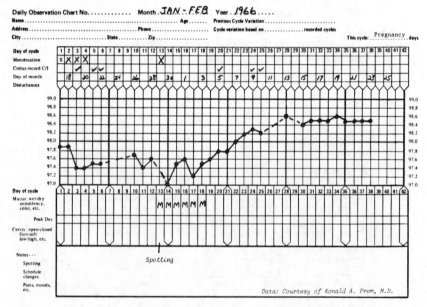

Figure 6.13c Coitus too Soon After Ovulation

Lack of Motivation, Misinterpretation or Not Following the Rules?

Sometimes it is difficult to say that any single factor led to an unplanned pregnancy, and such is the case with the experience expressed on the chart in fig. 6.14. The couple who submitted this chart at first felt that they had acted out of misinterpretation. Upon further reflection, they spoke of lack of motivation. However, at least one thing is clear: The basic rules were not followed, as the discussion below will make clear.

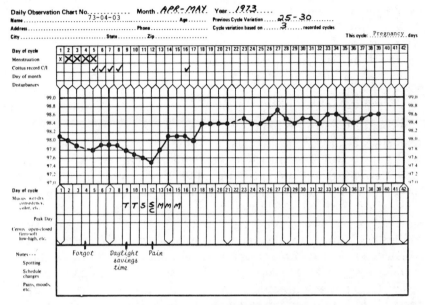

**Figure 6.14 Lack of Motivation,
Misinterpretation or not Following the Rules?**

1. Disregarding the 21-day Rule

It is the policy of the Couple to Couple League to recommend that a couple who are relatively inexperienced in natural family planning should not have coitus during the relatively infertile phase until they gain sufficient experience with the sympto-thermal method. After they have gained six months' experience, they can have coitus on the days allowed by the 21-day rule with relative security. The chart in fig. 6.14 indicates three immediately previous cycles, one of which was only 25 days long. The charting shows a disregard for the 21-day rule and the alternate-dry-days-only guideline.

2. Insufficient Mucus Observation

The sympto-thermal method calls for the recording of mucus observations every day past menstruation until the beginning of Phase III. No observations were recorded on days 6, 7, and 8. Perhaps one reason for this was that the woman thought that any vaginal discharge on these days was simply seminal residue rather than the beginning of the mucus symptom.

This illustrates the reason for the alternate-dry-days-only guideline: If a couple chooses to have coitus past the time indicated as relatively infertile by the 21-day rule, they should not have coitus on consecutive days.

If the woman's mucus notations are reliable, the rule "Peak + 4" would point toward day 16 as the beginning of Phase III. However, there is insufficient temperature corroboration at that point. The sympto-thermal interpretation would indicate day 18 as the first day of Phase III by Rule B.

3. Insufficient Temperature Rise

A significant error in interpretation was caused by regarding the three temperatures at 98.1° as the thermal shift. The high pre-ovulation level in this chart would be placed at 97.9°, and such a level would make it very apparent that the temperatures at 98.1° were not high enough. We have repeatedly said that the normal thermal shift is 4/10 to 6/10 of a degree; a rise of only 2/10 of a degree could be regarded as a thermal shift only when there was a long record of such experience. In this case, the history showed regular thermal shifts of 4/10 to 6/10 of a degree. The wife knew that her temperatures were not high enough yet, but the couple were no longer serious about postponing a pregnancy.

The temperature-only rule of three days of at least a 4/10 of a degree thermal shift would indicate day 20 as the beginning of Phase III; so also would the sympto-thermal Rule A; while the sympto-thermal Rule B and the five-day step-rise guideline would both indicate day 18. Coitus on day 16, as indicated in fig. 6.14, would be too early under any system looking for a basal temperature corroboration of ovulation.

4. Paying Too Much Attention to Insignificant Details

What allowed this couple to talk themselves into thinking that ovulation had occurred were two things. The wife felt a pain on day 12 that she associated with ovulation, and they apparently gave it primary importance, even though it should only have been used to corroborate other, more definite signs. Secondly, they paid attention to the temperature rise from the low dip on day 12 to the higher temperature on day 14. That particular shift is unimportant. What counts is the rise above the *high* level of the temperatures of the pre-ovulation phase (the pre-ovulation base).

This is in reality a happy chart. The husband was happy that his wife became pregnant, and she was glad that he was happy. And we are happy to have a chart that shows the importance of sticking to the rules and that is so instructive about several mistakes.

Conception probably occurred from the coitus between days 5 and 8, but it may have occurred from that on day 16.

Misinterpretation, Experienced Couple

The fall 1970 issue of *Coverline*, the quarterly publication of the Natural Family Planning Association of Connecticut, carried a discussion about the conception cycle illustrated in fig. 6.15. One comment saw it as possibly a "method failure," since intercourse on day 19 was apparently responsible for this pregnancy. However, using the principles advocated in this manual, there is no way in which day 19 could be considered the first day of postovulation infertility, and thus we must respectfully disagree. The comments below should make it evident that real emphasis on the mucus sign plus a normal requirement of a thermal shift of 4/10 of a degree do make a difference in interpretation.

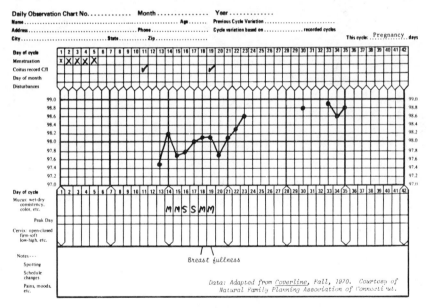

Figure 6.15 Misinterpretation By An Experienced Couple

First of all, this was an experienced couple who had used the basal temperature system successfully for years. Previous cycle variation ranged from 33 to 44 days. Perhaps because of these two factors, the woman did not begin recording temperatures until day 13.

Secondly, this couple did not follow the 4/10 of a degree rule. They estimated the pre-ovulation base at 97.8°. On that basis, the anticipated thermal shift level would be at least 98.2°. The first such temperature is found on day 22, whereas this couple indicate coitus on day 19.

Thirdly, the mucus notation system used here was developed prior to the current emphasis on the drying up of the mucus sign. Applying that rule retrospectively here, the last day of the fertile-type mucus might be anywhere from day 17 to day 19 (day 17 if the last day of "threads" is used as the peak; day 19 if day 20 was the first day of drying up). Thus, "Peak + 4" would yield anything from day 21 to day 23. Considering the fact that day 21 has not yet yielded a good temperature corroboration, we think a couple should wait for further evidence of the beginning of the postovulation infertility. If 97.8° is the pre-ovulation base, then Rule B would indicate day 23 as the first day of Phase III.

How did the couple who submitted this chart actually interpret it? The woman had a history of pre-ovulation rise (discussed in connection with earlier charts in this manual), and thus they discounted the rise on day 14, as we have likewise done. By establishing a pre-ovulation base of 97.8° and looking for three temperatures above it by only 2/10 of a degree (instead of a shift of 4/10 of a degree), they saw day 19 as the third day of elevated temperatures. In addition, the presence of only a few temperature recordings made it easy to err in establishing the pre-ovulation base. Finally, this occurred at a time, 1970, when much less emphasis was given to the mucus sign.

Pregnancy Apparently Resulting from Prolonged Sperm Survival

In this chart (fig. 6.16), we see a record of a cycle and sexual activity that resulted in pregnancy. The couple had previously calculated that day 8 was the last day of the relatively infertile phase, and they had sexual relations on the four days ending with day 8. The woman did not notice mucus until day 10. How did she become pregnant?

There are several possible explanations. Ovulation sometimes occurs several days before the temperature rise. If it occurred on day 10 or 11, it would have been within the usually accepted range of 72 hours for sperm survival. Another explanation would see ovulation occurring on day 12 or 13, thus entailing a sperm life of four or five days. The difficulty with both these explanations in terms of the data on the chart is that the chart does not indicate the presence of mucus until day 10, and the available evidence indicates that sperm life is quite short — a few hours to a day — in the absence of cervical mucus.

How, then, can we possibly account for this apparently extended sperm life? Our first explanation is sheer speculation, but perhaps coitus on four successive days created some conditions similar to mucus and aided sperm survival. The second and more likely explanation is that some mucus was already present on day 8 but was simply not observed. There would be, most likely, at least some residue of seminal fluid from the coitus the night before, and mucus secretion might have been mis-. understood to be simply the seminal discharge; the same would hold true of day 9.

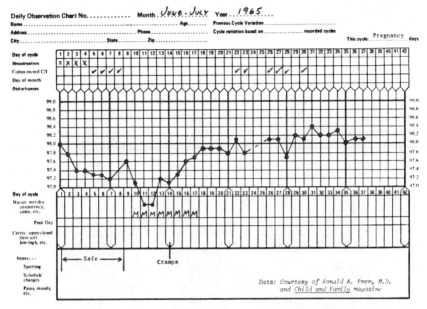

Figure 6.16 Apparent Long Sperm Survival

It should also be noted that this chart dates back to 1965. This was in the days when a 19-day rule was used for calculating the length of the relatively infertile phase, and experiences such as the one illustrated here led Dr. Prem to recommend the 21-day rule instead.

Pregnancies from Coitus During the Relatively Infertile Phase

These two charts serve to illustrate that the relatively infertile phase is only *relatively* infertile. The chart in fig. 6.17a shows coitus on days 7 and 8 and a resulting pregnancy. Let us try to reconstruct the thinking of this couple. Assuming that they were faithfully following the 19-day rule that was used in 1964 for determining the length of the relatively infertile phase, the shortest cycle previously recorded would have been 27 days (day 8 + 19 = 27). Further assuming that they were figuring on an average of 14 days between ovulation, they would have been anticipating ovulation no sooner than day 13 (27 - 14). However, in this fertility cycle, ovulation occurred most probably on day 10 or 11, thus unexpectedly early.

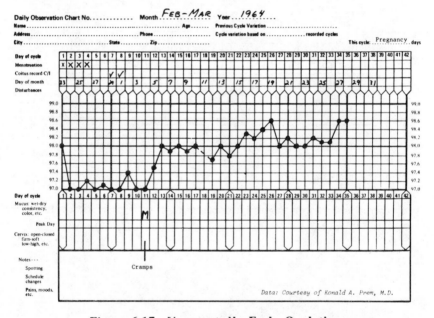

Figure 6.17a Unexpectedly Early Ovulation

The 21-day rule was developed partly as a result of such pregnancies; if it had been followed here, it is doubtful that pregnancy would have occurred.

The 1964 chart shows only one day of mucus, probably a day of heavy and very noticeable discharge. However, we think it must have been present also by day 8 in order to provide for sperm survival until day 10 or 11. The mucus on day 8 may have been obscured by the seminal residue from coitus the night before. This helps to illustrate the advisability of avoiding coitus on consecutive days in Phase I.

Fig. 6.17b shows coitus on day 6, the last day of menstruation, followed immediately by the mucus sign, a probable ovulation pain, and thermal shift. Most likely, cervical mucus was already present on day 6 but was obscured by the menstrual discharge. With mucus easily detected on days 7-10 and with ovulation probably occurring on day 8 or 9, pregnancy resulting from coitus on day 6 is readily explainable. Since this couple had designated day 6 as the last "safe" day under the 19-day rule, it is quite probable that conception would not have occurred if they had been following the 21-day rule. This chart indicates that while the days of heavy menstrual flow are infertile, the latter days of menstruation can be very fertile. Both charts show the value of the 21-day rule as contrasted with the 19-day rule used by the couples in these two cases.

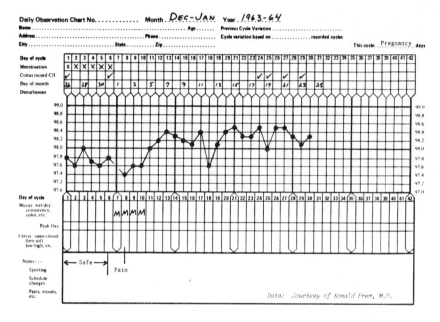

Figure 6.17b Fertility During Menstruation

An Unexplained Pregnancy?

The question mark in the caption for the chart in fig. 6.18 is very real. We are not sure whether this chart shows a pregnancy resulting from not following the rules or whether it illustrates a true method failure, meaning that the system failed to avoid a pregnancy for a couple who followed the rules.

The pre-ovulation high level in this case was 97.9°, as determined by the temperatures between days 5 and 11. Thus, we would be looking for a post-ovulation thermal shift to at least 98.3°. The coitus on day 27 was on only the second day of temperatures at the normally required 4/10 of a degree elevation. Thus, according to the three-day rule for elevated temperatures, we may say that this couple did not follow the rules.

However, if they were interpreting this as a slow rise and used the five-day rule, we would have to regard it as a method failure of the temperature-only system. All the qualifications for beginning the five-day count on day 23 and ending on day 27 were met: (1) the pre-ovulation base had been set by at least six temperatures; (2) the count did not begin until the temperature was actually at least 2/10 of a degree above the pre-ovulation high level; and (3) at least the last temperature was at the required 4/10 of a degree elevation (in this case, the last two

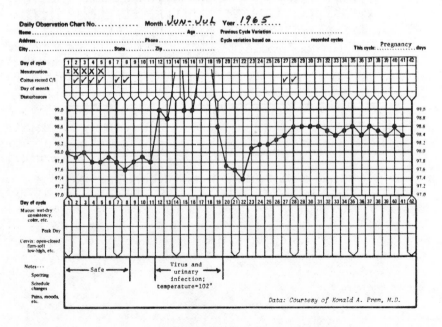

Figure 6.18 An Unexplained Pregnancy?

temperatures, on days 26 and 27, were at that level).

Thus, we must reiterate the caution of Dr. John Marshall with regard to the five-day rule of the temperature-only system: Where there are the most serious reasons to avoid pregnancy, don't use it.[16] Wait for the three temperatures at the required 4/10 of a degree elevation to indicate the beginning of post ovulation infertility. In this case, that would have meant waiting one more day.

When we first showed this chart at a Couple to Couple League meeting, two women came up immediately afterward and remarked that their experience with charting indicated that fever postponed the time of ovulation for them. We have not seen any research on this but pass on their experience, which may be helpful in similar situations.

Note also in this chart, which dates back to 1965, that the task of interpretation is not aided by mucus or cervix observations. Thus, this chart is not an example of a surprise pregnancy of the sympto-thermal method but of the temperature-only system.

Summary Comment on Surprise Pregnancies

One of the guiding principles of the Couple to Couple League is that every child — whether asked for or not — is a gift from God and is to be loved and respected for his or her own sake. As everyone knows, it has become a deadly custom in this country to kill many of the unplanned babies. We feel this has happened at least partly as a result of absolutizing the idea of the planned family and thus closing the mind and heart to the acceptance of the unplanned child. The acceptance of abortion did not just come upon the scene overnight; it grew out of some other ideas such as absolute personal freedom, absolute family planning, and a confusion of love with the pleasure of genital intercourse. However, many of us know from personal experience and many others know with a deep-down intuition that love is shown much more in the acceptance of adversity and difficulties for a good cause than by being self-willed; we know intuitively or have learned that pleasure and long-range happiness are by no means the same.

Thus, we have thought it appropriate to conclude a brief discussion of surprise pregnancies with a reminder that the value of family planning is only relative. What must be absolutized is the love we must have for all who enter our lives, whether at conception or as adults, whether we really invited that person or not. Planning says something about our anticipated response to an imagined future; our response to the present is the test of our love.

Section D. Special Situations

There are five situations that call for additional comment even if brief: (1) the anovulatory cycle; (2) the return of fertility after a miscarriage; (3) the loss of fertility during premenopause; (4) the return of fertility after discontinuing contraceptive pills; and (5) the return of fertility after childbirth (this will be discussed separately in Chapter 7).

The Anovulatory Cycle

The anovulatory cycle is one in which ovulation did not occur. Such cycles may occur occasionally during the fertile years of any woman. They occur more frequently in the premenopausal period, with some frequency in the first few postpartum menstrual cycles of the breast-feeding mother, and among women with certain endocrine disorders.

The chart in fig. 6.19 shows the pattern. This particular one came from a breast-feeding mother, but the temperature pattern would be similar for any anovulatory cycle.

Since there was no ovulation, there was no thermal shift. However, there may sometimes be the appearance of pre-ovulation mucus. The fact that there is no temperature rise after what may seem to be the mucus usually associated with ovulation indicates that ovulation did not occur.

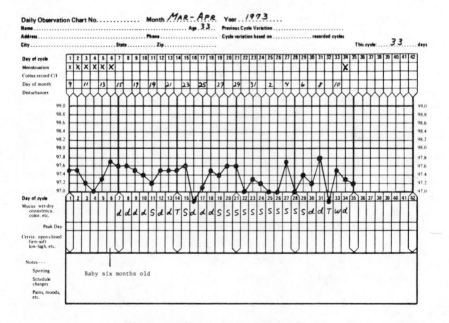

Figure 6.19 An Anovulatory Cycle

What about coitus during an anovulatory cycle? Rather obviously, coitus could be engaged in on any day in the cycle without the possibility of conception when there is no ovulation, but such knowledge is of little help because a cycle cannot be determined anovulatory until the next menstrual period. Those who wish to postpone coitus until after the basal temperatures have clearly indicated ovulation and the beginning of post ovulation infertility will have no such indication and will therefore not have coitus during that cycle.

The anovulatory cycle points to the definite advantage of observing the pre-ovulation signs of mucus and cervix. The couple who are experienced in the observation and interpretation of these signs may follow the guidelines for these signs and have coitus accordingly (that is, the fourth dry day after the mucus sign and/or the fourth day of the cervix closing, if it had opened). In the cycle in fig. 6.19, the mucus rule of thumb would have yielded day 10 as the last day available for coitus since the cycle had no four-day sequences of dry days after the appearance of the fertile type of mucus indicated by the "S" symbol on the chart. Most anovulatory cycles would have many more dry days; this chart shows that the return of fertility after childbirth is probably near at hand.

Special attention is drawn to the fact that if more than one appearance of pre-ovulation mucus occurs, the guidelines for refraining from coitus must be followed each time.

Also, coitus should be avoided during any vaginal bloody discharge not preceded by a thermal shift because it cannot be determined with certainty whether such discharge is an anovulatory menstruation or the usually lighter breakthrough bleeding discussed previously (fig. 6.7).

The Return of Fertility After Miscarriage

The time after a miscarriage is almost always fertile. Temperature records should be begun immediately after the miscarriage. In some cases, the temperature will remain high for some time (as it was during pregnancy) before it drops to the usual pre-ovulation levels. Couples who desire to postpone another pregnancy should refrain from coitus until postovulation infertility has been definitely indicated by the sympto-thermal signs of mucus and basal temperatures.

Couples who desire another pregnancy immediately may attempt to achieve it during this first post-miscarriage cycle.

124

The Premenopausal Period

When a woman approaches menopause, or change of life, she will frequently experience irregularity even if she has had a history of regularity during her fertile years. The irregularity may be of three types.

1. Length of Cycle

Menstrual periods that may have occurred at regular 28-to-33-day intervals may now begin occurring at 45, 60, or 90-day intervals but without any particular pattern. Sometimes a woman may think she has had her life's last period after six months without menstruation and then have a menstrual bleeding. With this type of irregularity, it is advisable to use the mucus and cervix observations regularly because they indicate the approach or presence of fertility. One experienced woman reported that the cervix observation was by far the most helpful sign during her premenopausal years.

2. Non-fertile Cycles

During premenopause a woman may experience menstruation that has not been preceded by ovulation. These are called anovulatory or non-fertile cycles. Because no ovulation has occurred, there will be no temperature signs of ovulation although there may be the appearance and disappearance of cervical mucus (see preceding pages for further comment on the anovulatory cycle).

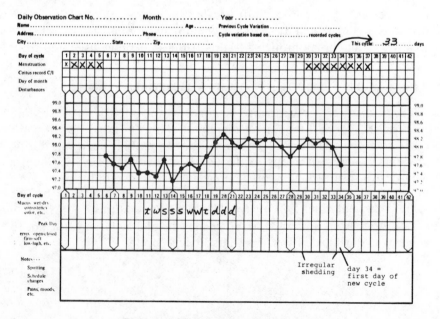

Figure 6.20 Irregular Shedding

3. Irregular Shedding

During the premenopausal years there is an increased possibility that a woman will experience the onset of menstruation while the temperature is still elevated (fig. 6.20). The temperature may remain elevated for several days after menstruation begins and drop to pre-ovulatory levels only near or at the end of the menstrual flow. This may cause some problems in using the 21-day rule. When this situation occurs, the first day of the new cycle should not be taken as the first day of menstruation but the first day of temperature drop. Irregular shedding always develops into a menstrual period; it does not leave only to have a menstrual flow appear sometime later.

Coming Off the Pill

The oral contraceptives used in the 1960s were generally of a stronger dosage than those used in the 1970s, some of which are called low-dosage pills or the Minipill. By way of review, it should be recalled that the typical oral contraceptives achieve their effectiveness by a triple mechanism: suppression of ovulation, changes in the cervical mucus to render it hostile to sperm, and changes in the endometrium (the lining of the uterus) to make it hostile to the implantation of a newly conceived human being (at the blastocyst stage of development).

The high-dosage pills were thought to achieve their effectiveness primarily through suppression of ovulation although it has been reported that ovulation still occurs from 2 to 10 percent of the time in women taking the Pill.[17] Opinion seems to be divided about the lower-dosage Pill, and of course there are significant differences in the types of Pill, dosage, etc. However, there seems to be a consensus that the lower-dosage pills are less likely to suppress ovulation and thus more likely to rely on one or both of the other mechanisms to prevent pregnancy or its continuation.

We must emphasize that whenever a drug (or a device such as the IUD) prevents the continuation of the newly conceived life by preventing implantation in the uterus, it has not acted as a contraceptive but as an abortifacient. The persons responsible for its use are thus responsible for the killing of a newly conceived human being. Perhaps the realization of this accounts for the many women who want to "get off the Pill" and begin planning their families the natural way.

A woman coming off the Pill may experience some irregularities that she will normally not experience once her body is on a natural cycle again. Sometimes, temperatures will be very erratic for one or more cycles. Sometimes, the mucus secretion will be quite heavy almost all

126

the time for a few cycles; it may well be that her body has stored up excess estrogen from the Pill and that it is taking several months to return to normal. Sometimes, the first cycle is fertile; sometimes, it isn't. Sometimes, a woman will have several more or less "regular" cycles followed by one that is either very short or very long. In short, because of the variety of the drugs used and the variety of effects they have upon different women, it is very difficult for us to make many generalizations about "typical" experiences of coming off the Pill apart from saying that it may take a little time before normality is reestablished. Rarely, menstruation may be postponed for months or even years.

Nevertheless, we have included three charts. In the cycles immediately off the Pill, we will tend to emphasize the temperature more than the mucus because the mucus might still be affected by residues from the Pill. (See "Just-off-the-Pill" guideline in Section A of this chapter.)

The two cycles charted in fig. 6.21a and 6.21b came from the same woman in her first two cycles off the Pill. In the first cycle, the mucus pattern is of no help, especially to an unexperienced woman. However, the series of low temperatures from day 22 to day 29 establish a pre-ovulation base of 97.2°. The temperature pattern on days 30-32 is ambiguous, but a clear thermal shift is established by the recordings for days 33-35. Phase III has certainly begun by the evening of day 35. The cycle continues off the chart for a total of 43 days.

The second cycle shows how both mucus and temperature signs are more normal a month later. The mucus is apparently less abundant and even disappears some days after ovulation. However, it is still of little help in determining the beginning of postovulation infertility in this cycle. The pre-ovulation temperature base is easily set at 97.5°, thus setting the thermal shift level at 97.9°. The five day post-pill temperature-only guideline establishes day 25 as the beginning of Phase III.

The cycle in fig. 6.21c was likewise a first cycle off the Pill. It is included here simply to show that some women have clearly defined patterns right away. With the pre-ovulation base established at 97.1°, both the temperature and mucus signs coincide to indicate day 24 as the beginning of postovulation infertility. However, CCL would still recommend a day 25 interpretation according to the 5 day post-pill guideline.

It is not an uncommon experience among natural family planning counselors to find that couples just coming off the Pill sometimes experience difficulties in the adjustment of their sexual activity as well as in the interpretation of what is happening physiologically. Because sex is so greatly psychological and because our sexual attitudes are so all-important in the regulation of sexual activity, perhaps it might be helpful at this point to review some thoughts that can influence our attitudes.

Coming off the Pill (Figure 6.21)

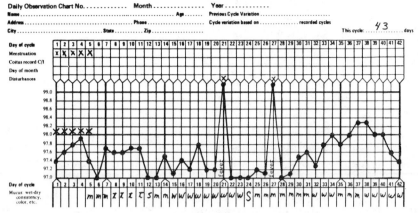

Figure 6.21a

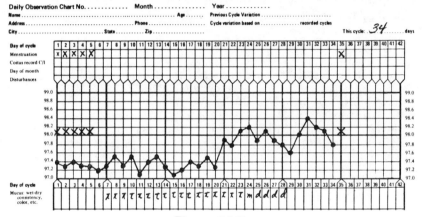

Figure 6.21b

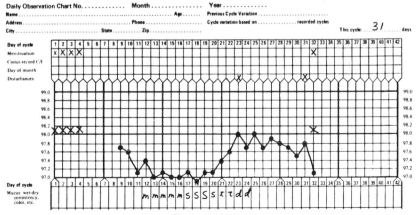

Figure 6.21 c

Those who think in terms of nature and ecology might reflect on the fact that the contraceptive drugs and devices have done a certain violence to nature. They know that any violence against nature calls for some sort of restoration and that this always comes at a price, usually at the price of some form of self-control. Those who think in the psychological terms of maturity certainly know that maturity does not come automatically with age but only at the price of growing pains. This is also true of sexual maturity and the growth in self-control needed for mature sexuality. Those who think in moral terms and have come to regard the practice of contraception as unethical know that their past mistakes or sins call for some sort of penance or work of reconciliation with God and nature. Those who think in Christian religious terms can see in the suffering of Christ something that gives meaning to their own difficulties or sufferings in the effort to be faithful to him. In the last analysis, almost any difficulties can be borne if they can be seen as meaningful, and the above brief thoughts were intended to offer various meanings that can enrich the process and pain of human growth.

References

[1]Josef Roetzer, "Erweiterte Basaltemperaturmessung und Empfangnisregelung," *Archiv fur Gynakologie* 206 (1968), 195-214.

[2]John Marshall, *The Infertile Period* (Baltimore: Helicon Press, 1969), p. 86.

[3]Maureen Ball, "A prospective field trial of the 'ovulation method' of avoiding conception." Europ. J. Obstet. Gynec. Reprod Biol, 6/2, 63-66.

[4]Hanna Klaus, M.D. et al. "Behavioral Components Influencing Use Effectiveness of Family Planning by Prediction of Ovulation (Billings Method.)" *The Family.* 4th Int. Congr. of Psychosomatic Obstetrics and Gynecology, Tel Aviv, 1974 (Basel: Karger, 1975) pp. 218-221.

[5]John Marshall, "Cervical-Mucus and Basal Body-Temperature Method of Regulating Births: Field Trial." *The Lancet.* August 7, 1976, pp. 282-283.

[6]B. Vincent et al., *Methode therminque et contraception: Approaches medicale et psycho-sociologique.* (Paris:Masson, 1967) pp. 52-73.

[7]J. Marshall. *The Infertile Period,* p. 42, refers to the late Dr. Holt, who devised a system of windows using this "cross" principle for the interpretation of charts. Fortunately, most of this has been made unnecessary by the sympto-thermal system of fertility awareness with its use of the mucus and cervix signs along with temperatures.

[8]ibid., p. 71.

[9]*The Infertile Period.*

[10]ibid., p. 30.

[11]ibid., pp. 30-35.

[12]ibid., p. 30.

[13]ibid., p. 35.

[14]Vincent, op. cit.

[15]Referred to in Marshall, op. cit., p. 111.

[16]Marshall, op. cit., p. 35.

[17]John Peel and Malcoln Potts, *Textbook of Contraceptive Practice* (New York: Cambridge University Press, 1969), p. 99.

Notes

Notes

7

The Return of Fertility
After Childbirth

Most studies on natural family planning have given relatively little attention to the return of fertility after childbirth. To put it more precisely, emphasis has been given to the bottle-feeding mother and the quick return of fertility. Breast-feeding has generally been discouraged, and the general advice has been to wean quickly so as to get back to regular menstrual cycles. Such studies, however, do acknowledge in a sort of backhanded way that there is real difference in the return of postpartum fertility between the bottle-feeding mother and the breast-feeding mother. What is usually overlooked are the significant differences between the various types of breast-feeding and how these differences affect the return of postpartum fertility. Accordingly, in this chapter we discuss four distinctly different situations and how the return of fertility after childbirth is affected by each. By far the greatest emphasis will be given to what we call ecological breast-feeding for several reasons. First of all, we would like to encourage this form of baby care because of all its benefits for both baby and mother; secondly, this form of baby care raises questions in people's minds and we hope to answer a few of them; thirdly, most of the time only this ecological breast-feeding has any significant effect as far as a long period of postpartum natural infertility is concerned.

Preliminary Remarks About Childbirth

However, before we discuss the various forms of baby care and the related return of fertility, we think it might be worthwhile to say something about the weeks immediately before and after childbirth. Some husbands become impatient for the resumption of coitus after childbirth because they feel they have gone a long time without it. What we have said previously about attitudes is relevant here, but it is also true that in many cases couples have been advised to refrain from coitus for reasons that have nothing to do with fertility, personal character development or health. The advice is routinely given by some doctors under the guise of health reasons that the couple should refrain from coitus for six weeks or more before the anticipated delivery and for six weeks following childbirth. Add a week or so for the typical late delivery, and we have a routine "doctor's order" to avoid coitus for a quarter of a year. Certainly situations may arise in any marriage where the couple may have a good reason to refrain from coitus for much longer periods. Our problem is that the typical routine medical advice about refraining from coitus for that twelve or thirteen week period before and after a normal pregnancy is simply not at all necessary. If the wife is having a normal, healthy pregnancy and the husband has no venereal disease or other infection in the genital area, the advice to refrain from coitus for six weeks prior to the anticipated delivery is unfounded. The more appropriate advice would be to tell such a couple that there are no medical reasons to refrain from coitus prior to the beginning of labor. Their decision to engage in or refrain from coitus would have to be based on other considerations such as the wife's comfort, personal discipline, and so forth.

After childbirth, the appropriate advice to the medically healthy couple would be to refrain from coitus until the wife would feel comfortable. The idea of waiting until after the six weeks' checkup may be necessary in cases where the woman had difficulty with the healing of the episiotomy, but it is not a universal necessity. A woman can receive individual counseling on this matter from her physician, who can tailor his advice to her particular condition. Women who have a prepared and natural childbirth and who completely breast-feed may be in shape weeks before those who participate in the cultural customs of medicated childbirth and bottle-feeding.

We write this on the strength of statements made by Konald Prem, M.D., professor of obstetrics and gynecology at the University of Minnesota Medical School. If your doctor disagrees, politely ask him for the medical evidence that contradicts what we have written. We also encourage couples to read "The Cultural Warping of Childbirth" by Doris Haire, a well-documented study and commentary on childbirth practices.[1]

Interestingly enough, many of the same doctors who routinely prescribe twelve or thirteen weeks of sexual continence become quite anxious to prescribe a contraceptive or sterilization when the couple have decided to refrain from coitus for two or three weeks for reasons of natural family planning. With increasing frequency we have been hearing of physicians who have introduced the subject of sterilization to their patients. We think that the institution of marriage, the institution of medicine, and society as a whole will be much better off when physicians learn how to help people to live within the natural order and limit their practice of medicine to the attempted cure and prevention of disease. The unnecessary removal and destruction of medically healthy organs for supposedly personalistic and sociological reasons has been followed by the much more grievous evil of the unnecessary removal and destruction of innocent, unborn babies from their mother's womb—for those same supposedly personalistic and sociological reasons.

We intend no polemic against the medical profession; certainly, there are still doctors, hopefully many, who regard the natural as the norm and the goal, who limit their practice of medicine to the cure and prevention of disease, and who do not regard pregnancy, even the unplanned pregnancy, as a disease. However, the tone that is evident in these paragraphs has developed not out of any initial prejudice but rather out of hearing many personal accounts of what is happening today. We hope things will change; we think that a well-informed patient-clientele is one of the best ways of reforming some of the ills in the current practice of medicine. To such persons we would offer this word: simply, politely, but firmly ask for the medical evidence. Do not make the assumption that competence in treating disease in any way carries with it a competence as a moralist or spiritual advisor—or even a special competence in knowing how to foster the natural.

The Bottle-feeding Mother

Fertility generally returns quite soon after childbirth for the woman who bottle-feeds. As with most things in nature, there is some variation but a general pattern prevails. The earliest ovulation that has been detected after childbirth has been at 27 days postpartum.[2] This would mean that menstruation would occur at approximately 41 days postpartum unless Phase III is short, as sometimes occurs in the first few cycles postpartum. Such cases of ovulatory cycles in the first six weeks postpartum are infrequent; the available evidence indicates that when the first postpartum menstruation occurs at 42 days there is only about a 5 percent chance that it has been preceded by ovulation.[3] In other words, in about 95 percent of cases, when menstruation occurs at six weeks postpartum it was not preceded by fertility.

During the first three weeks postpartum, as the above evidence suggests, there is almost no possibility of conception. Any coitus during this time would be dependent upon the woman's health and comfort. By the fourth week, we are already within the range of recorded fertility. Thus, the practical advice for avoiding another pregnancy immediately for the bottle-feeding mother would be as follows.

1. Begin taking basal temperatures at least by day 14 after childbirth. Refrain from coitus (or genital contact) from childbirth until the temperature records have given a very definite indication of the return

of postovulation infertility.

2. The wife can attempt to make the observations of cervical mucus once the bloody discharge within the weeks right after childbirth has disappeared. However, such observations may be impractical for detecting pre-ovulation mucus with a number of bottle-feeding mothers because the extended duration of postpartum bloody vaginal discharge may obscure the observation of mucus.

If there are no other vaginal discharges and if the woman is experienced in making the mucus observation, then the couple may engage in coitus on the mucus dry days prior to the first menstruation, but *not* on consecutive days. However, it should be kept in mind that this period is only relatively infertile and carries a slightly higher degree of fertility than the postovulation infertility, as has been made clear from the material in Chapters 3 and 6.

Since the majority of bottle-feeding mothers probably experience six weeks or more of postpartum discharges, the most common practice will be to refrain from coitus until after the first menstruation.

3. Beginning with the first menstruation, the couple should regard themselves as back in the regular fertility cycle. Sometimes the second menstruation will occur without a preceding ovulation, but this would be relatively uncommon in the bottle-feeding mother; between the second and third menstruation it would be quite rare for such a mother not to have ovulated. Thus, after the first menstruation, the couple should use the regular rules of natural family planning for fertility awareness and the regulation of their practice of coitus or genital contact.

Breast-feeding Plus Supplements

Almost all the confusion that exists about breast-feeding and postpartum infertility is due to the practice of partial breast-feeding plus supplements. This is what we call "token breast-feeding" or "cultural breast-feeding." Later in this chapter we explain what is meant by ecological breast-feeding as contrasted with this token or cultural breast-feeding. It is ecological breast-feeding that is associated with an extended period of postpartum natural infertility.

Therefore, for all practical purposes, the mother who, during the first 6 months, supplements breast-feeding with formulas, baby foods, juices or other liquids including water, cereals or other solids must regard herself as a bottle-feeding mother. The same holds true for nursing mothers who use pacifiers, who breast-feed according to a schedule, who go for long periods between nursings and so forth. These are the common forms of cultural breast-feeding that tend to restrict the baby's frequent nursing at the mother's breast.

For anything less than full ecological breast-feeding, it is quite common for fertility to return quickly after childbirth, frequently just as soon as for the mother who does not breast-feed at all. Thus, the guidelines for the bottle-feeding mother should be applied in all the various forms of cultural or token breast-feeding, that is, in all cases that do not meet the criteria for full ecological breast-feeding. Quite simply, one cannot expect the natural benefits of any ecological relationship unless the requirements for that relationship are fulfilled.

Complete Breast-feeding with Deliberate Weaning

By deliberate weaning we mean the stopping of nursing over a very short period of time. The effect on the return of ovulation is the same whether the baby is weaned in a day or over a period of a week. However, weaning in a period of a day or two can be extremely uncomfortable for the mother because her milk supply may continue to be ample for several days, thus giving her engorged breasts. Quick weaning is often hard on babies, and we would encourage parents who do wean the baby off the breast to continue to hold and cuddle the baby often, especially during his feeding times.

In his practice, Dr. Konald Prem has successfully used the following guidelines for a ten-day weaning program for the mother who wishes to nurse for only three or four months.

1. The mother should be totally breast-feeding before the ten-day weaning program begins.

2. Beginning with day 1 of weaning, the couple may continue to have coitus until day 10, by which time weaning should be completed. They should begin to take temperatures, if they have not done so already, by day 1 of weaning.

3. On day 11 after the beginning of weaning the couple should regard themselves as fertile and should refrain from coitus if they do not desire an immediate pregnancy.

4. The couple should continue to refrain from coitus and any genital contact until the thermal shift with three days of sufficiently elevated temperatures, which indicates postovulation infertility.

We would add, of course, that if the mucus or cervix signs indicated the return of fertility prior to the beginning of weaning or between days 1 and 10 of the weaning process, such signs should be interpreted as indicating an unexpectedly early return of fertility.

Such a deliberate weaning program may be followed up through the fourth month of total breast-feeding. Beginning with the fifth month, even the ecologically breast-feeding mother may occasionally experience the return of fertility and should be on the lookout for the various signs of fertility.

Furthermore, it should be recognized that such a ten-day weaning program is no assurance of a quick return of fertility. We have seen charts that have indicated a fairly long time between the end of the short weaning period and the return of fertility.

What about the woman who fully breast-feeds for a shorter time, say three to six weeks, and then either weans completely or introduces supplements? In the case where the fully breast-feeding mother weans completely over a ten-day period at any time during the first three or four months, the guidelines in this section would be applicable.

However, if she goes from ecological breast-feeding to cultural or token breast-feeding at any time, then the earlier comments about the bottle-feeding mother and the mother who supplements her breast-feeding are applicable.

Ecological Breast-feeding

This section deals with what may be the most controversial part of this book for some because the subject of ecological breast-feeding goes far beyond the subject of natural family planning. In fact, because breast-feeding a baby is so much more than "birth control" we would never recommend that a mother breast-feed her baby just for that reason. It is important to do the right things for the right reason, and the right reason for breast-feeding is that it is the best for the baby—nutritionally, dentally, medically, emotionally, and any other way you can think of.

However, when a mother begins to think in terms of what is really best for her baby and realizes that it is ecological breast-feeding, then she has a problem: Our society does not expect a mother to experience truly natural mothering. How can she explain to well-meaning relatives and friends that natural, ecological breast-feeding really *does* space babies? How can she explain to a well-intentioned but poorly informed mother or mother-in-law (or pediatrician for that matter) that her baby is not starving just on breast milk but is getting the best food he can get?

Since breast-feeding is so much more than natural child spacing, and there is so much satisfaction in it for the mother, she will very often want to follow the natural pattern of letting the baby wean at his or her own pace, which may be months after the return of fertility. Can she find any support for nursing a baby who can walk, even one who can talk, in a culture in which most women won't breast-feed at all and in which it is not common to nurse beyond six months?

It is not within the scope of this book to reply fully to such questions, which merely indicate the full context of breast-feeding and natural mothering. It is not even within the scope of this book to document in any thorough way the statement that ecological breast-feeding spaces babies or to explain in any detail how to achieve the practice of ecological breast-feeding in the face of all our cultural customs to the contrary. The questions we have touched on are among the many related topics that really are the subject of another book, a companion to this, *Breast-feeding and Natural Child Spacing: The Ecology of Natural Mothering.*[4] The many letters we have received lead us to believe that men and women who are interested in breast-feeding, child spacing, and natural mothering will enjoy it and benefit from reading it.

Because of the many questions that have been raised about ecological breast-feeding and the return of fertility, we thought it best to adopt a question-and-answer format in the rest of this section. For purposes of keeping the pronouns simple, we will treat the baby as a boy.

What is ecological breast-feeding?

Ecological breast-feeding is the type of nursing that respects and follows the natural order; it avoids practices that would upset the balance of nature between mother and baby. In this balance, the baby receives the best nourishment physically and emotionally, and the mother normally receives an extended period of natural infertility and absence from menstruation. In addition, the mother receives satisfaction and fulfillment in her womanly role of mothering.

How does it extend the period of infertility?

Research indicates that the infant's frequent sucking at his mother's breast helps to suppress ovulation.

Can breast-feeding affect the birth rate?

Sometimes a striking example is helpful. Dr. Otto Schaefer, writing in the November-December 1971 issue of *Nutrition Today,*[5] noted that the Eskimos' birth rate increased 50 percent as they moved into or near towns and adopted the practice of bottle-feeding. The newer crop of babies likewise had more health problems since they have been deprived of their best food—mother's milk. Away from the influence of urbanization, Eskimo mothers breast-fed from two to four years, with babies arriving about three years apart.

In another study (1969-1971), Dr. Schaefer and Dr. J. A. Hildes noted that the Igloolik Eskimo mothers who nursed traditionally conceived twenty to thirty months after childbirth, whereas the younger mothers who were now exposed to "cultural" practices were conceiving two to four months after childbirth. [6]

You don't have to be an Eskimo to have the breast-feeding advantage of natural infertility, but you do have to be courageous enough to go against our cultural customs. There is a mother-baby ecology that is destroyed by cultural practices, but it is easy to learn the rules of this ecology.

What are the basic rules for ecological breast-feeding?

You simply follow these do's and don'ts. The thing to remember is that frequent sucking at the breast is the key to ecological breast-feeding.

1. Do let your baby nurse as often as he wants. Don't set up a nursing schedule of so many feedings a day. Don't set a limit for the time at each breast. Since breast milk is so much easier for baby to digest than bottle milk and since the baby enjoys pacification at the breast, it is quite natural for your breast-fed baby to nurse often.

2. Don't aim for your baby to sleep all through the night. It is the frequent and regular sucking that suppresses ovulation, and eight to twelve hours without a nursing may be too long. Put your baby to breast before you go to sleep; if he wakes up during the night, bring him to bed with you and let him nurse while you and he sleep. Sleeping with baby, besides its emotional benefits for both mother and baby, is an extremely important factor in natural spacing. It is at these times (during naps or during the night with mother) that baby will suck often and contentedly to satisfy his needs.

3. Don't use a pacifier. The breast is a wonderful mothering tool and the best pacifier for your baby. Sucking at the breast has a calming effect upon the infant, and a tired baby falls asleep easily at the breast. This mothering aspect of breast-feeding is extremely important to the emotional well-being of baby and likewise plays an important part in the natural spacing mechanism.

4. Don't give him any solids, liquids, juices, cereals, or water during his early months. His only source of nourishment should be your milk until he's big enough to begin grabbing food off the table and stuffing it into his mouth. An older baby is also ready for solids when at about six months of age he begins to swallow a small amount of food when it is offered instead of pushing it out of his mouth. Some babies will want solids at five months of age, and others are not ready until a few months later.

5. Don't force weaning. Natural weaning occurs gradually and usually over a period of many months or a few years at baby's pace—not society's.

6. Do be one with your baby. Avoid situations which separate the two of you.

7. Do be prepared to debate with your baby's doctor and some well-meaning but misinformed friends and relatives. Let the doctor check your baby's blood if he questions the baby's iron supply at a certain age. Studies and observations show that anemia in the "totally" breast-fed baby up to six months of age is extremely rare.[7] In the rare case where iron is required, iron drops can be used until the baby is ready for solids. This iron test is very simple, requiring only a drop of blood from

baby's finger. It helps to remember that the average doctor learned very little about breast-feeding and child spacing in medical school and that his own wife probably used bottles. Therefore, some doctors are not very helpful when it comes to breast-feeding.

Increasing medical evidence today shows the dangers of overfeeding babies, and it relates the early introduction of solids, liquids, and formulas to the increased amount of allergies and chronic ear infections, increased hospitalization of babies, increased incidence of intestinal diseases and anemia, and so on.[8] Nature's food is still superior. In those early months of life it is good to know that the mother alone can provide her baby with the very best.

8. Attend La Leche League meetings if available in your area, or write the nearest League representative for any information or questions you would like answered. The best source of information (in addition to their monthly meetings) is their excellent breast-feeding manual, *The Womanly Art of Breast-feeding*.[9] La Leche League has over 2,000 groups in the United States and fourteen foreign countries. This nondenominational "mothering" group offers the expectant or nursing mother proper information and support with regard to breast-feeding and natural mothering. Even mothers with successful nursing experience in the past have benefited from attendance at these meetings.

9. Don't be discouraged if your relatives and friends think you are an oddball. Instead, reach for the support that you can find in La Leche League, in the Couple to Couple League, and in the previously mentioned book *Breast-feeding and Natural Child Spacing*. [10]

Can any mother nurse?

In the briefest terms, yes; any normal woman can nurse. However, the ignorance and misinformation about breast-feeding in a bottle-feeding culture have led many women to think that they could not nurse successfully.

Many mothers who once felt strongly that they would be unable to nurse and others who gave up trying to nurse previous babies have discovered through La Leche League meetings that their reasons were invalid and have gone on to nurse their next baby with relative ease. We know of individual mothers who were told by their doctors that they couldn't nurse because of their milk, their blood, their medication, or their physical condition. These mothers, however, learned later that they could nurse. Many of them found the support they needed from La Leche League. We always recommend that any mother who is interested in nursing keep in touch with La Leche League, and if anyone tells her to wean—no matter what the reason— to contact a League representative or the League medical advisory board first, especially when she still desires to have this nursing relationship with her child.

Any woman can nurse, but no woman should nurse while taking any form of the birth control Pill, including the Minipill. The Pill may decrease or dry up the mother's milk supply, and the artificial hormones may affect the baby through the mother's milk.

Does ecological breast-feeding save money?

Yes. We might mention the costs of departing from the natural ways of doing things, namely, departing from ecological breast-feeding. At first, we might tend to think only of the immediate expenses. Here, we would find that the cost of bottles, formulas, and baby foods probably runs about $200 in the first six months, thus giving that much of a savings to the properly breast-feeding mother.

In addition, the breast-fed baby is normally healthier than the bottle-fed baby. He will have fewer allergies, fewer chronic ear infections, fewer intestinal diseases, and more built-in immunities. For example, one study showed that bottle-fed youngsters had eleven times more hospital admissions during the first ten years of life than breast-fed children.[11]

Breast-fed children will typically have fewer dental problems. In areas where prolonged nursing is common, thumbsucking does not seem to be a problem among older children. Likewise, nursing stimulates the growth of the whole facial area; thus, the incidence of orthodontic cases among cultures where women nurse for several years is much lower than the high incidence noted here in the United States.[12] Breast-feeding is recommended as a preventive measure against tongue thrusting, a frequent dental problem associated with bottle-feeding. [13] Studies have showed that the dental decay rate was lower in breast-fed children. [14] Many formulas have sugar added, and this sugar may do serious harm to baby's teeth. In short, nature's plan provides better health for your youngster, and better health means fewer medical and dental expenses.

Is the natural infertility ecology more delicate for some women than for others?

Yes. For many women this natural spacing process is a delicate matter. For example, the mother who lets her baby sleep in a separate bed and soon finds that he is sleeping all through the night may find her periods returning. The mother who uses the pacifier or who gives her baby early solids or an occasional bottle may find her periods returning.

Sometimes a mother who leaves her baby with sitters or who relies on "mother substitutes" (for example, *excessive* use of swing chairs, infant seats, playpens, cribs, etc.) may find her periods returning early because these have lessened the baby's sucking at the breast. Nature is usually generous to the mother who is generous and unselfish in meeting her child's emotional and nutritional needs. Nature intended that the mother and baby have a close "oneness" in their relationship. Thus, *physical closeness between mother and baby* could be said to be an important aspect of natural spacing. The mothers who follow this pattern for the first time and give nothing but total love to their baby find joys and rewards that they never experienced with their other children. Mothers who interfere with this "oneness" or with nature's plan may find menstruation right around the corner.

There are also those mothers at the other end of the scale who require very little stimulation to hold back their menstrual periods. Some may give only two good nursings a day and still not have a return of menstruation. Some mothers may also use a pacifier or leave the baby with sitters occasionally or not encourage night feedings and still they experience a lengthy absence of periods. Even these mothers would probably experience a much lengthier amenorrhea if they followed the natural mothering program. Some mothers who desire another baby and who have had a long absence of periods become anxious for their cycles to return in anticipation of another desired pregnancy. However, these mothers generally enjoy waiting on nature and would not consider weaning abruptly for their own interests when the child still needs this nursing relationship.

How long will this natural infertility last?
In a study conducted by the authors, the mothers in the United States who followed the natural mothering program outlined in *Breast-feeding and Natural Child Spacing* and in the preceding pages of this manual averaged 14.6 months without any menstrual bleeding or periods following childbirth. Individuals, of course, varied from that average. We found four mothers who had an early menses return before nine months postpartum — one as early as six weeks. We also had a few who experienced no periods for two years due to nursing; one experienced her first period thirty months after childbirth. The most frequent return of menstruation occurred within thirteen to sixteen months following childbirth. Considering the cultural influences in our society today, we feel this study is significant because it shows that American mothers who are serious about breast-feeding can experience a natural infertility similar to that of nursing mothers in other parts of the world who are not affected by artificial child-care practices.[15]

If mothers appreciate the mothering aspects of breast-feeding and follow the guidelines given in this chapter, both they and their babies will generally be healthier, and most of these mothers will experience an extended period of natural infertility. Generally speaking, those couples who desire a spacing of eighteen to thirty months between the births of their children will find breast-feeding sufficient for natural family planning. This, of course, is said only with reference to those who follow the "natural mothering" program.

Does the sex of the baby influence the return of menstruation?

No. Some mothers have told us that they felt they had a lengthy absence of periods while nursing because they had a boy baby (they did not have the same experience with their breast-fed girl babies). On the other hand, some mothers have said that they felt this long absence from menstruation was due to the fact that they were nursing a girl baby. *The important factor is how often and how much a baby nurses,* and that is influenced mostly by mothering practices.

Which comes first for the nursing mother — ovulation or menstruation?

Most women who follow the natural mothering program of total breast-feeding and gradual weaning will experience menstruation before the first postpartum ovulation. However, the available evidence indicates that about 6 percent of fully breast-feeding mothers practicing no form of fertility awareness or birth control have become pregnant prior to their first postpartum menstrual period.[16] A greater percentage ovulate but do not become pregnant for various reasons. Partial or token breast-feeders have a higher chance of becoming pregnant prior to the return of menstruation.

What is the risk of becoming pregnant while nursing?

After the first menstruation, there is soon as good a chance of pregnancy as at any other time during the fertile years. For practical purposes, we are ignoring the fact that the nursing mother *may* have a second or a third infertile menstrual cycle. Once menstruation has returned, a woman should regard herself as probably fertile. *Before* the first menstrual period, the evidence suggests that the mother who follows the ecological breast-feeding policy of this manual has approximately a 5 to 6 percent chance of becoming pregnant as indicated above.

However, during the time she is engaged in total breast-feeding — in other words, during a typical first five or six months — the risk of pregnancy is even smaller, closer to 1 percent than to 5, before the first post-partum period.

Can other methods of natural family planning reduce the risk?

Figure 7.1 shows a case in which the signs of ovulation gave ample indication of the return of fertility to this experienced woman. In this chart, the small letters indicate small quantities of mucus. Note that there was a long period of mucus that was small in quantity and not accompanied by any significant opening of the cervix. Note also that this woman was in her fifteenth month since childbirth and that the chart shows the return of ovulation and her first menstruation. It is not unusual for nursing mothers to have an extended period of some form of mucus prior to the return of their first ovulation. Some women may even experience mucus during one or more anovulatory cycles before ovulation eventually resumes.

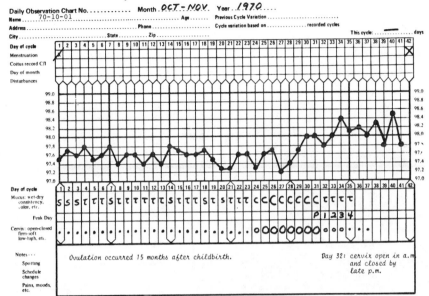

Figure 7.1 Nursing Mother: Detection of Ovulation Before First Menstruation After Childbirth.

Note also, however, that the presence of the mucus that is clear and with threads (indicated by the large "C's") is accompanied by a very definite opening of the cervix. The temperature graph points up the value of the other signs of ovulation in the total interpretation. Some people might be tempted to regard day 32 on this chart as the third day of temperature elevation, but the very experienced mother who sent us the chart is quite convinced that ovulation occurred on day 32.

For one thing, day 32 is *not* the third day of temperature elevation. Rather, day 32 had dipped to 97.8°, only 1/10 of a degree above the readings of days 26 and 29. Sustained temperature rise means that the temperature has stayed up without dipping to the pre-ovulation lower pattern.

Secondly, on what appeared to be a couple of days of rise, days 30 and 31, there was much clear and stringy mucus, and the cervix was open. Thirdly, the temperatures on those days are only 3/10 of a degree higher than the pre-ovulation base of 97.7°, while the normal thermal shift is 4/10 to 6/10 of a degree.

Lastly, this woman was convinced from her own past experience that her cervix began to close up on the day of ovulation. Thus, we would say that day 36 on this chart would be the first safe day by Rule C for the couple who were serious about avoiding pregnancy. Rule B would indicate day 35.

Can an inexperienced woman detect the signs of returning fertility while nursing?

We cannot make the generalization that *every* inexperienced woman will observe these signs. However, we do have evidence that inexperienced women *can* detect them. The cervical mucus is usually quite abundant when it appears during amenorrhea prior to the return of the reproductive cycles. Women who have a difficult time observing mucus in later cycles generally find this observation very easy to observe prior to the first menstrual period. Some women may note much wetness instead of clear, stretchy mucus, and this too is an important sign of possible approaching fertility or menstruation.

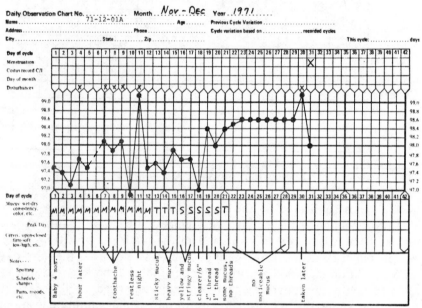

Figure 7.2 Fertile First Menstrual Period Post-partum: Detection by Inexperienced Woman

The woman who submitted the chart in fig. 7.2 had learned about the Couple to Couple League just a few weeks before the first temperature recorded here. She had had no previous experience in making mucus observations. In fact, she questioned whether she would be able to use this sign, as she felt she had mucus all the time during regular cycles. When her baby was four months old, she observed what she thought was the presence of mucus. She wondered if this was the kind of mucus she was looking for and had a *knowledgeable* physician examine her. The doctor helped her to identify the thick and sticky mucus then present and advised her to refrain from relations with her husband. Five days later the mucus was clear and would stretch six inches. The next day her temperature rose and 2 days later (day 21) the mucus began to disappear. Thirteen days after the six-inch mucus, her menstruation returned.

This chart shows the importance of making the mucus observations and temperature recordings even while fully breast-feeding, especially if menstruation had returned early during previous nursing, as it had for this woman who nursed her baby often, day and night. By observing the mucus she became aware that fertility might be approaching, and by taking her temperature she had assurance that ovulation had definitely occurred. We stress the importance of temperature recording in this case because sometimes a breast-feeding mother will experience quite a long period of mucus before her first menstrual period.

After the first fertile menstruation, will the cycles show exact regularity?

Not necessarily. This chart (fig. 7.3) records the second postpartum cycle from the same woman who submitted the previous chart (fig. 7.2). It shows a long period of mucus extending from day 21 through day 40. Thereafter, the temperatures remained elevated at 98.6° until the end of the cycle, day 48. Long cycles such as this are not uncommon among nursing mothers right after the first postpartum menstrual period, and they tend to return to normal within a few cycles.

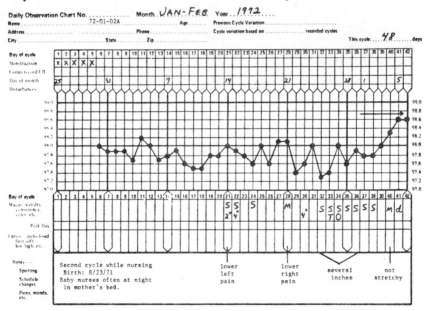

Figure 7.3 Extended Period of Mucus

It should be noted that even though this mother began introducing solid food to her baby during the weeks covered by this chart, the baby still continued to nurse very frequently, thus providing the sucking stimulus that acts to inhibit ovulation. This mother, however, is an exception to our breast-feeding program. Her history shows an early return of menstruation with previous nursing babies — usually at about 7 or 8 months postpartum. This was the earliest postpartum return of her menstrual cycle.

The observations were made on the basis of the mucus discharge on underclothes and external genitalia rather than by internal examination, and that may account for the absence of some recordings (e.g. on days 20, 23, 29, 31).

Since the temperature remained high for more than eight days, it is fairly certain that this was a fertile, ovulatory cycle. If the couple had been relying solely on external mucus observations, and days 25, 26, and 27 were regarded as "dry days," they might have resumed relations on day 28, calling it the fourth day beyond the peak of day 24. This would have been risky at best. The temperature, however, remained low.

Ovulation probably occurred between days 36 and 39, and we believe that a chart such as this confirms the Couple to Couple League policy of advising couples to use at least two ovulation signs which complement each other.

Can you have more than one infertile menstrual cycle while nursing?
In fig. 7.4 we have a case of a woman who was very definitely engaged in ecological breast-feeding. Still, her first menstruation occurred at four and a half months postpartum. She then experienced two definitely anovulatory cycles (January-March and March-April). In the third cycle postpartum, there was a thermal shift indicative of ovulation, but the extremely short duration of elevated temperatures (three days) may indicate an infertile ovulation. Cycle 4 postpartum was anovulatory; cycle 5 was questionable. Cycles 6 and 7 seem to indicate infertile ovulations; cycle 8 indicates a fertile ovulatory cycle; cycle 9 is questionable; and cycles 10, 11, and 12 indicate fertile ovulatory cycles. Throughout the year covered by this sequence of charts, the baby continued to nurse regularly day and night. Note also how the cycles tended to become more regular beginning with the fourth cycle postpartum.

Note also that the cycles are shorter than usual because of a short Phase III. This is typical for nursing mothers during the early postpartum cycles. For example, in the ninth cycle after childbirth this woman ovulated about day 17 and menstruated on day 26. Normally with a 25-day cycle, ovulation would occur earlier in the cycle. Thus, after weaning is completed, this woman may use the 21-day rule with reference to her non-nursing cycles. She would not have to use this 25-day cycle as her shortest cycle. In a regular cycle if she ovulated on day 17, her menstrual period would appear around day 30 or shortly thereafter.

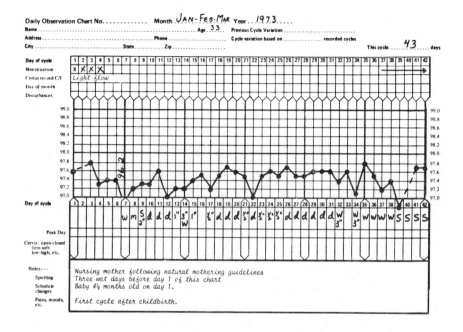

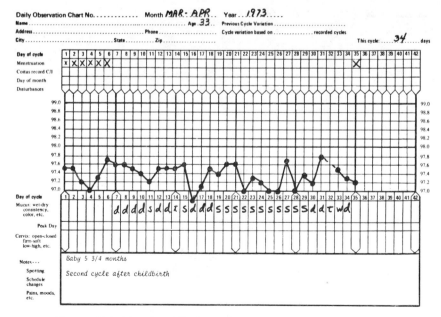

Figure 7.4: Nursing Mother: First 12 Cycles After the Return of Menstruation

(page 1 of 6)

148

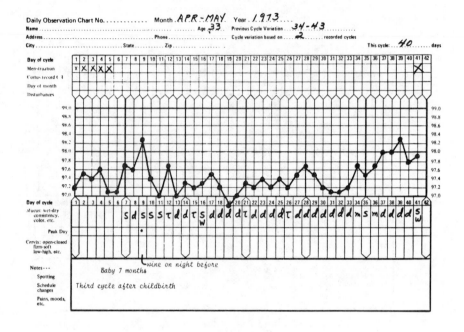

Daily Observation Chart No. . . . . Month *APR-MAY*. Year *1973*
Name . . . . Age *33* Previous Cycle Variation *34-43*
Address . . . . Phone . . . . Cycle variation based on *2* . . . . recorded cycles
City . . . . State . . . . Zip . . . . This cycle: *40* . . days

wine on night before

Baby 7 months

Third cycle after childbirth

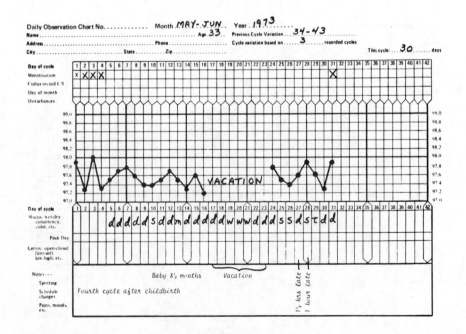

Daily Observation Chart No. . . . . Month *MAY-JUN*. Year *1973*
Name . . . . Age *33* Previous Cycle Variation *34-43*
Address . . . . Phone . . . . Cycle variation based on *3* . . . . recorded cycles
City . . . . State . . . . Zip . . . . This cycle: *30* . . days

VACATION

Baby 8½ months *Vacation*

Fourth cycle after childbirth

½ hrs late
1 hour late

Figure 7.4 (page 2 of 6)

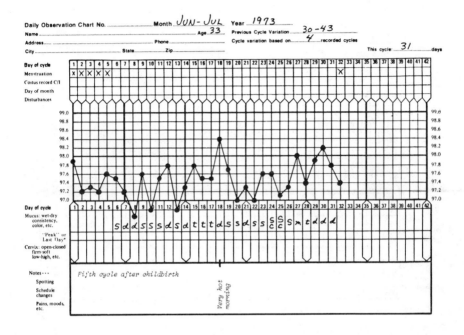

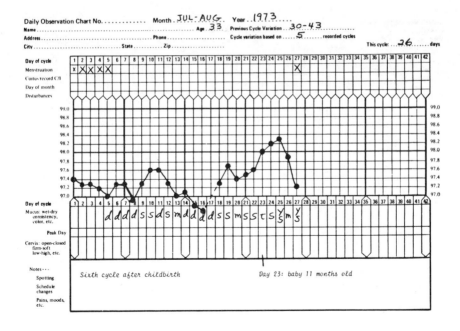

Figure 7.4 (page 3 of 6)

150

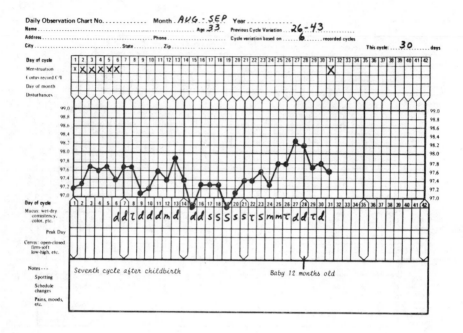

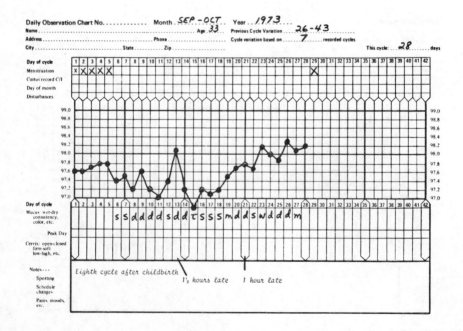

Figure 7.4 (page 4 of 6)

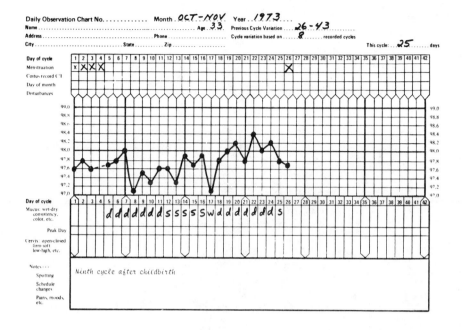

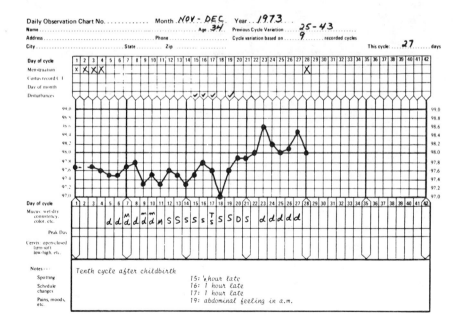

Figure 7.4 (page 5 of 6)

152

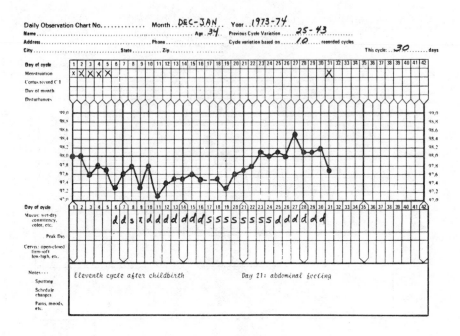

Daily Observation Chart No. .... Month .. DEC-JAN .. Year .. 1973-74
Name .... Age . 34. Previous Cycle Variation ... 25-43
Address .... Phone .... Cycle variation based on ..... 1.0 .... recorded cycles
City .... State .... Zip .... This cycle: ... 30 .... days

Notes···
Eleventh cycle after childbirth   Day 21: abdominal feeling

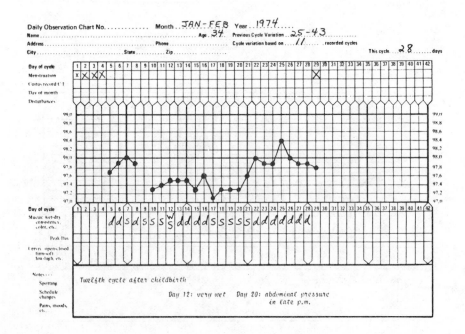

Daily Observation Chart No. .... Month .. JAN-FEB .. Year .. 1974
Name .... Age . 34. Previous Cycle Variation ... 25-43
Address .... Phone .... Cycle variation based on ..... 11 .... recorded cycles
City .... State .... Zip .... This cycle: ... 28 .... days

Notes···
Twelfth cycle after childbirth
          Day 12: very wet   Day 20: abdominal pressure
                                      in late p.m.

Figure 7.4 (page 6 of 6)

When should the nursing mother begin taking basal temperature?

Temperature readings should be begun when any of the following occur:

(a.) introduction of solids or liquids;

(b.) any sudden decrease in sucking (due to sickness, etc.)

(c.) menstruation or spotting, no matter how slight;

(d.) the appearance of cervical mucus;

(e.) six months postpartum.

Temperatures taken before any of the above indications will provide a good history and a good base for the first pre-ovulation levels. Also, in the event of a surprise pregnancy, they will indicate when it occurred. Typically, the basal temperatures for the nursing mother tend to be erratic and somewhat lower than usual. Because of the somewhat erratic temperature patterns and our desire not to cause unnecessary concern, it is not a Couple to Couple League policy to make into a natural family planning rule the practice of taking temperatures before any of the above indications.

How should a nursing mother regard the mucus that may last for a considerable time?

The safest thing to do is to regard it as a sign of fertility and to refrain from intercourse. However some women experience certain types of mucus for some time before they are actually fertile as in fig. 7.1. It should be noted that nursing mothers may observe an abundance of mucus two to four weeks before their first menstruation even when there is no ovulation. Some mothers will note that they have blotches of mucus on and off. These appearances of mucus may have no resemblance to the mucus that indicates fertility, and thus they may be of no concern *if* the mother is well informed and experienced in the mucus observation. The less experienced mother should have no genital contact on these days or for three days following the appearance of wet or clear, stretchy mucus. The couple should also be watching for a thermal shift, but even if no thermal shift occurs and if she is dry for three days, then relations may be resumed on the fourth day. They should regard themselves as in an extended Phase I and not have coitus on consecutive days.

More research is needed on the connection between fertility and the various types of mucus. At this time we can only say that the couple in which the woman is well experienced in the observations of mucus and cervix may decide to allow coitus where the less experienced couple may decide to refrain.

As noted repeatedly, the available research indicates that about 6 percent of nursing mothers practicing no form of fertility awareness become pregnant before their first menstruation after childbirth. The preceding paragraphs have been intended to help nursing mothers reduce further that small risk of pregnancy. Further research may improve fertility awareness in the postpartum, premenstrual phase. However, continence on the days of possible fertility indicated by accurate observation and interpretation of the mucus and cervix signs should yield results as good as those attained by couples having coitus only on nonconsecutive dry days beyond the limits of the 21-day rule during normal fertile cycles. Couples who postpone coitus until after the sympto-thermal indications of being in Phase III—the postovulation, absolutely infertile phase—will have almost no risk of pregnancy, but they may have a very long wait.

Once menstruation returns, can it be suppressed again?

Yes, for some mothers, especially in the early months. We have recorded cases of menstruation being suppressed from one month postpartum to sixteen months. In some cases (especially in the early months postpartum), the cycles can be suppressed for many months. In other cases, ovulation may be delayed within a cycle; this long cycle may give the appearance of having missed a period. These situations occur for different reasons. Common reasons are (1) a child's illness with resulting increased nursing, (2) a mother's change in mothering which increased the nursing, or (3) special circumstances which increase or decrease the nursing.

An example of one such circumstance might be a family's move from one place to another. The effect upon the child may be such that he increases his nursing for a few days or weeks. In another special circumstance, family gatherings on holidays or a vacation away from home can result in decreased nursing. In these situations, the mother may feel restricted when being around those who do not have favorable attitudes toward breast-feeding. Her period returns within a few weeks due to limited nursing during the time spent with relatives or friends. (This latter situation is unfortunate because normally trips to strange places and among strange people should continue to suppress the cycles, as babies usually require more nursing for emotional reasons when exposed to a new situation.) Once the mother reestablishes her old nursing pattern, she may find her periods are suppressed once again. Some mothers have had a regular period one month postpartum but then have had no periods for many months. In some cases, a hospital environment which greatly restricts nursing immediately from birth could be a factor for an early return of menstruation before the cycles are once again inhibited.

There are mothers, however, who will experience their first period soon after childbirth and will attempt to suppress their cycles once again by nursing more often but will still continue to have their periods.

Are there any general recommendations for nursing mothers who are interested in the natural mothering program that haven't been mentioned yet?

Yes. The nursing mother should eat nutritionally balanced meals and get lots of rest during the night (which she can do if she is sleeping with the baby) and even a short or long nap during the day. A woman who does excessive work around the house or continues to have a heavy, demanding schedule may find her milk supply has decreased. This influence on the milk supply may mean a return of her periods.

Is something wrong with the mother's body if she has a lengthy absence from menstrual periods while nursing?

No, there is nothing wrong with her body. This condition is a healthy, normal situation for the nursing mother. It helps her regain her strength after pregnancy and childbirth by not losing part of her iron supply through periodic menstruation.

We have met quite a few nursing mothers who have gone back to their doctors for a pap smear and find that the doctor is concerned that they haven't had a period for some twenty months. Some doctors suspect pregnancy, tell the mother to wean, and then administer a pill for a few days which will supposedly cause a "period" *if* she is not pregnant. Fortunately, under our self-awareness system the woman would know whether she was pregnant or not. Secondly, the pill may not bring on a "period" when the woman is not pregnant. In one such case, the woman followed her doctor's advice. She weaned her baby and took the pill for three days. When she had no "period" within two weeks of taking the pill, her doctor said on two different occasions that she was pregnant. She disagreed. About six weeks from the date of weaning, she noticed fertile-type mucus and had a well-defined thermal shift. If she had believed her doctor and resumed relations, this woman possibly could have become pregnant and the approximate time of conception would not have been accurately known. It is an old story that assuming pregnancy results in pregnancy.

Will menstrual periods be regular while nursing?

No hard-and-fast answers can be given. Generally speaking, the woman who follows our natural mothering program will have her periods return much later than the token breast-feeder. The nursing mother frequently has several longer cycles and then settles into her regular pattern.

What causes spotting?

Any treatment such as a pap smear or cauterization can cause spotting or considerable bleeding for a few days. This is related to the treatment and not to the menstrual cycle.

The normal type of spotting seems to indicate that ovulation and regular menstruation may be just around the corner. The spotting may occur for only one or two days, or it may occur on and off for one or two weeks.

We know of a few women who have become pregnant within a short time after the first spotting. Therefore, any spotting—no matter how slight—may be a sign that fertility or menstruation is returning. If the woman is not already doing so, she should begin making mucus observations and recording temperatures.

A woman who has extensive, prolonged spotting should see her doctor.

Can a mother nurse during menstruation or throughout pregnancy?

Yes, there is no reason to wean because of menstruation or pregnancy. Mothers have nursed through an entire pregnancy and have given birth to healthy babies. In our culture, it is commonly thought that a woman should wean during early pregnancy. We know of women who have weaned due to a pregnancy but then later had a miscarriage or a stillborn baby; they sadly regretted their decision to wean. One mother noted the difference between the child that had been weaned during pregnancy and the child that nursed throughout pregnancy. The weaned child was very hostile towards the new baby, but the nursing child accepted the baby and remained a very happy toddler after being displaced from the breast. She felt this was an added bonus to prolonged nursing.

Sometimes weaning occurs naturally during pregnancy; the mother finds nursing uncomfortable due to tender breasts or hormonal changes in her body, or the child appears not to like the taste of milk during pregnancy or the colostrum, which develops in the latter months of pregnancy.

When the mother follows the recommended natural mothering pattern, when should the couple refrain from coitus?

We assume that this couple are very serious about avoiding another pregnancy. We have no single answer, but the following comments may be helpful in determining the periods of infertility.

1. The earliest that ovulation has been detected in the non-nursing mother was twenty seven days after childbirth.[17] It is thought that the *fully nursing* mother will always have a later return of ovulation.

2. For the fully nursing mother, ovulation (and thus fertility) before the tenth or twelfth week is very rare. However, after the first menstrual period or with the beginning of mucus, the couple who are serious about avoiding pregnancy should assume that fertility has returned.

3. When the baby begins taking solids, there is probably some increase in the possibility of fertility returning soon even though the mother continues regular nursing.

4. Ovulation will normally be preceded by a noticeable mucus discharge. (See figure 7.1) (We think we could say "always" but we said "normally" to take into account some medical quirk.) As we have said several times before, observation of this mucus should give ample warning time that fertility is returning. When examination reveals the presence of mucus, especially when its quality ranges from creamy-thick to the stretchy, raw-egg-white type or when it gives a feeling of vaginal wetness or slipperiness, the couple should certainly refrain from genital contact if pregnancy is not desired.

Are there sometimes fairly long periods of refraining from coitus when the wife is following the program of ecological breast-feeding and baby-led weaning?

For the couple who are extremely serious about avoiding another pregnancy, there can be some fairly long periods of refraining from coitus because of uncertainty about possible fertility, especially during the time of transition from breast-feeding amenorrhea and infertility to the resumption of regular cycles. For example, a breast-feeding mother may have a menstrual period and then go for well over a month before ovulating. If a couple had decided to wait until the beginning of Phase III, they may have an extended period of coital abstinence.

Or, for another example, a woman may have extended periods of mucus. It may not be the fertile type associated with ovulation, but the couple may not be willing to risk a mistake in judgment about the type of mucus, especially if she is inexperienced in this observation.

In such cases, some couples may choose to accept the slight risk of pregnancy inherent in using the mucus guidelines during Phase I; they may learn to make use of the dry days between patches of mucus, always waiting until the fourth day of dryness after any fertile-type mucus. Other couples may choose to refrain from coitus until there are definite signs of being in Phase III.

If the couple choose the more conservative course, will such coital abstinence affect their marriage?

Some people think that any extended abstinence will adversely affect a marriage, and some think that *other* couples will refuse a course of action that entails some sexual self-control even if they themselves will accept it. Thus, some have routinely encouraged early weaning in the hopes of establishing regular cycles soon after childbirth.

It is our opinion and experience that couples are willing and able to accept some lengthy periods of coital continence if they have sufficient motivation (e.g., putting the baby's need before theirs) and keep up their noncoital means of communicating love and affection. In fact, the marital relationship, far from being adversely affected, can actually be improved during periods of extended coital continence, as is indicated by the following letter from a reader.

The baby had a bout of pneumonia in early December. She had to be put in the hospital for a time. My good doctor got us a private room so I could stay with her. Molly, however, went on a nursing strike and after we got home things began to happen. We noticed all sorts of signs pointing to menstruation and although Molly started breast-feeding when we got home I got my period about six weeks later. We did pretty well though—Molly was then 11¾ months old. We are following the manual like a bible. We are now in a cycle and no signs of anything! Temps show nothing and there has been very little mucus. Thus far we have abstained for ten weeks—I do hope I get that second period! Actually all is going very well and I am wondering if we are abnormal: it isn't bothering us. In fact, we are closer than ever before.

On the other hand, other couples may weigh the various factors and decide to wean their baby so that cycles may return to a pattern uninfluenced by nursing. In such cases, a 10 day weaning period may be more comfortable for both mother and baby. When the baby is older than four months, fertility should be assumed from the beginning of the weaning phase although some experienced women may choose to rely upon cervix and mucus signs as the indicators of fertility.

With so much emphasis placed on natural mothering and breast-feeding where does the husband fit in?

The husband is of particular value to the nursing relationship in providing support and love to both wife and baby. In addition, while the wife is experiencing a deeply satisfying relationship with the baby, she must also remember that her husband still needs to know that he's very special. Deepened communication and extra signs of marital love and affection should be present between husband and wife so that the husband does not feel neglected and does not feel that time his wife spends with the baby is time not spent on him.

A mature husband will appreciate the benefits of the nursing relationship and will be proud that his wife is giving *their* baby the very best care. Furthermore, he should be sharing in parenthood by cuddling and holding the baby. Such caring for his child's needs will help to make him more aware both of the time involved and the satisfaction that can be gained by relating to and enjoying his baby.

Is there any connection between childbirth practices and natural family planning?

Yes, problems with breast-feeding can sometimes be traced to the type of childbirth, and these can lead a mother to abandon the attempt, thus losing the typical period of breast-feeding infertility. For example, a medicated delivery can leave the newborn baby drugged and unable to get off to a good nursing start; and a good start can make the difference in some cases. In addition, separation of mother and baby at the hospital can interfere with the early establishment of a satisfactory nursing relationship.

Summary of natural mothering, breastfeeding and
child spacing program

Basic Principles:

1) The sucking stimulation by the baby at the breast when repetitious and frequent inhibits the menstrual cycles.

2) Natural mothering almost always provides this adequate stimulation. By natural mothering we mean that type of baby care which follows the natural ecology of the mother-baby relationship. It avoids the use of artifacts and follows the baby-initiated patterns. It is characterized by the items in Phase I and II below.

PHASE I of Natural Mothering: "MOTHER ONLY"

This phase usually produces infertility as long as the package is complete. What's in the package?

—Use of the breast for pacification
—Frequent nursing
—Sleeping with or near baby (night feedings)
—Absence of schedules
—Absence of bottles or pacifiers or early cups
—Absence of any practice which tends to restrict nursing or separate mother and baby
—Total breastfeeding in the early months

PHASE II of Natural Mothering: "MOTHER PLUS OTHER SOURCES"

—Begins when baby starts solids from the regular meal table. Liquids are begun later, again when baby begins on his own.
—Continues over a period of a year or two or more until baby gradually loses interest in nursing.
—Includes what may be a long period when the baby will be nursing as much for emotional reasons as for nutrition.

Phase II is a very gradual program in which the amount of nursing is 1) not decreased at all at first and 2) lessened only gradually at baby's pace. For the majority of mothers, Phase II will be longer than Phase I with regard to natural infertility **if** the natural mothering program is followed. Our survey indicated an average of 14 1/2 months of amenorrhea for mothers following this form of mothering.

Risk of Pregnancy: Under the natural mothering program there is about a 1% chance of pregnancy occurring before the first menstruation during the "mother-only" phase assuming regular coitus and no form of birth control. Once the baby begins solids and other liquids, there is about a 6% chance of pregnancy occurring before the first menstruation. The Couple to Couple League helps mothers to reduce this risk by teaching them to observe the mucus and cervical signs which occur before ovulation.

Natural Spacing by Breastfeeding Alone: For those couples who desire 18-30 months between the births of their children, "natural mothering" should be sufficient.

References

[1]Doris Haire, "The Cultural Warping of Childbirth, *ICEA News,* (Spring 1972). This booklet is available through the International Childbirth Education Association: 1414 N.W. 85th Street, Seattle, Wash. 98117.

[2]T. J. Cronin, "Influence of Lactation upon Ovulation," *Lancet* 2 (1968), pp. 422.

[3]Konald Prem, "Post-Partum Ovulation." Paper presented at La Leche League International Convention, Chicago, July 1971.

[4]Sheila Kippley, *Breast-feeding and Natural Child Spacing: The Ecology of Natural Mothering,* (New York: Harper & Row, 1974; Penguin paperback, 1975). Available through CCL as well as at most bookstores.

[5]Otto Schaefer, "When the Eskimo Comes to Town," *Nutrition Today* (November-December 1971), pp. 15-16.

[6]J. A. Hildes and O. Schaefer, "Health of Igloolik Eskimos and Changes with Urbanization." Paper presented at the Circumpolar Health Symposium, Oulu, Finland, June 1971.

[7]*Anemia: Rare in Breastfed Babies.* This pamphlet is available from the La Leche League, Franklin Park, Illinois.

[9]For the lay person we recommend Dr. Richard Applebaum's book *Abreast of the Times,* which is available only through the La Leche League and the International Childbirth Education Association. For the medical professional we recommend the following booklet: D. B. Jelliffe and E. F. P. Jelliffe, "The Uniqueness of Human Milk," *The American Journal of Clinical Nutrition,* 24 (August 1971), p. 1019.

[9]This breast-feeding manual is available through La Leche League.

[10]Kippley, op. cit.

[11]Robbins E. Kimball, "How I get Mothers to Breast-feed," *Physicians Management* (June 1968).

[12]Mary White, "Breast-feeding: First Step Toward Preventive Dentistry," *La Leche League News,* July-August, 1972, p. 57.

[13]Daniel Garliner, *Your Swallow: An Aid to Dental Health.* Pamphlet. The Gulf Building, Suite 715, 95 Merrick Way, Coral Gables, Florida.

[14]White, op. cit.

[15]S. K. Kippley and J. F. Kippley, "The Relation Between Breast-feeding and Amenorrhea: Report of a Survey," *JOGN Nursing,* (November-December 1972), pp. 15-21.

[16]Prem, op. cit.

[17]Cronin, op. cit.

Notes

Notes

8

Questions of Morality

Just as Chapter 2 could only touch on the religious dimension of questions that arise about family planning, so also our comments here can scarcely begin to touch on the moral values in this issue. Certainly, a single chapter is no place to attempt an analysis to which entire books have been dedicated. However, the reader may find it helpful to have something written about the common questions that keep coming up.

One of the most frequent questions is usually stated something like this: "If contraception and natural family planning both have the same objective of avoiding pregnancy, how can there be any moral difference between them?" Sometimes, no question is even asked and people bluntly state that it doesn't make any difference which method you use if the end purpose is the same. Such a statement fails to stand up under thoughtful investigation. If somebody wants my car, it makes a great deal of difference what "means" he uses to get it — whether he buys it from me or steals it. If a particular married couple want more money so that they can live in a bigger house, it makes all the difference in the world how they get it — whether they engage in the dope trade (which might get them into that house in a hurry) or whether they try to cut expenses and save (which might never get them into their dream house). In each of these cases, the purpose has been the same but there is a great moral difference in the ways and means of accomplishing it.

Does this also hold true about the various ways and means of family planning? If a person says "no," then he or she is saying that any means of family planning is morally permissible because the end is the same. We think that most readers will reject the killing of the unborn child as a method of family planning, no matter how widely practiced this is in China, Japan, Scandinavia, and in the English-speaking countries as well. At any rate, whoever rejects the killing of the unborn as a morally valid means of family planning accepts the principle that the end does not justify the means and that not all the ways of family planning are morally equal.

Another common question concerns the morality of particular

methods of contraception. We have already seen that the IUD is not really a method of contraceptive family planning but rather is an abortifacient means of family planning. The moral judgment that has to be placed on this is the same as for surgical abortion, and it would also hold true for the "morning-after Pill' and the "once-a-month Pill," which flush out the uterus. The use of surgical abortion, the IUD as a mechanical abortifacient, and these abortifacient drugs all have similar function — the preventing of the *continuation* of pregnancy by the killing of the developing but unborn child. The moral term for such premeditated killing of the innocent is murder.

The right-to-life movement and the reaction against it have made it clear that the pro-abortionists who admit that abortion is killing a young human being still reject calling the act murder. They insist that such a term can only be applied where there is malice involved in the killing. Such a criterion would prevent us from calling Hitler, Eichmann, and Stalin murderers because we cannot prove malice on their part, and thus we think it is a criterion without value. To be guilty of the moral crime of murder, it is sufficient to realize that one is killing a helpless and innocent human being, one who has in no way lost his or her personal right of continued existence.

We have already seen that the drugs usually referred to as the Pill operate in somewhat ambiguous and different ways. Some most likely suppress ovulation, others may also act as spermicides, but they all apparently affect the lining of the uterus so as to prevent implantation should conception occur. When conception occurs but implantation is prevented, these drugs have acted as abortifacients rather than contraceptives. We have also noted that there are certain hazards to personal health associated with these drugs. Thus, the moral question about the Pill is actually twofold.

Is it morally permissible to take a drug that may act as an abortifacient and that may also do serious harm to the mother when the desired birth regulation could be effected by less drastic means? Suppose the issue concerned a weight control pill. The same question could be asked: Would it be morally permissible to take a weight control drug that might cause an abortion or seriously injure the woman's health when the desired weight loss could be accomplished by less drastic means? The answer in this case is obvious. It would be immoral because it is wrong to endanger one life unless it is unavoidable in the effort to save another life; it is likewise wrong to endanger one's own life or health except for very serious reasons, especially when less dangerous alternatives are available. What holds true for a weight control pill is equally valid when applied to a birth control drug. This is especially true when there are other means of birth control that carry no risk of being abortifacient and that also entail no risk to the woman's health. Therefore, it is bad medicine and bad medical ethics to prescribe the Pill. This would be clearly recognized by all in the case of the weight control pill, but there are strong forces that work toward diminished moral vision when it comes to birth control.

The next question that usually arises notes that the previous criticisms of various forms of birth control have been based on the moral consideration that these forms have attacked the values of human life and health. But what if a couple used means that were unquestionably "only contraceptive" such as the condom, diaphragm, and the practice of coitus interruptus? This, of course, is the question that has been raised in the religious debate on this issue, and it might be rephrased in this way: Does the practice of contraception within marriage affect the meaning of the marital sex act, the very meaning and the value of the coital embrace, the meaning and the value of marriage itself?

This is the most difficult question to answer because it involves three related but not identical mysteries of life: the mystery of love, the mystery of marriage, and the mystery of sex. We call them mysteries because no matter how much you talk about these aspects of life, no matter how much you read, study, meditate, think, and pray about them, no matter how much you write about them, you know that the thoughts of others and yourself have still not adequately explained these realities. Anyone who attempts to address the morality of any of the modern questions about sex, whether it be premarital relations, group marriages, simultaneous or serial polygamy, homosexuality, contraception, etc., is faced with these related mysteries of life. Still, the human mind that asks these questions also tries to answer them, however incompletely.

Rather obviously, many people have said that marital contraception does not adversely affect the meaning of marriage, sex, and love. This is not the place for a detailed analysis of the pro-contraceptive arguments, but a few lines may help readers to understand why many people have not found their arguments attractive.

1. The "can do" argument. This approach says that since man's mind has figured out *how* to practice artificial contraception, therefore he can (morally) do it. Some bring God into the picture by saying that God gave us brains and expects us to use the products of our brainpower. This argument is really amazing, since it would likewise apply to atom bombs, instruments of torture, drug peddling, etc. The ability to do something, no matter how clever, is simply no guarantee that it is morally right to do it.

2. The "man can't do it" argument. This approach says that man and woman are so weak and the sexual urge so huge that it is impossible for them to refrain from coitus in the face of desire. The Bible has a more optimistic view of man and woman; as already mentioned, the Jewish law forbade coitus for twelve days beginning with menstruation. The

words of God that come to St. Paul as he sought the alleviation of some temptation, "My grace is sufficient for you" (2 Corinthians 12:9), also contributes to the inability to accept the pessimistic view of man that is enshrined in this viewpoint.

3. The "lesser of two evils" argument. This approach grants that contraception is an evil because it directly opposes the order of creation. However, this argument runs, it is a greater evil not to have coitus if the married couple think they need it for their marital happiness. This approach is similar to the previous one and is very closely related to the argument about ends and means; it also tends to incorporate the view that frequent, regular coitus is an absolute necessity for a happy marriage. The evidence on marital unhappiness despite unlimited contraceptive sex plus the very positive experiences of many couples practicing natural family planning leads many to think that this approach is erroneous and based on a very inadequate view of man, woman, love, sex, and marriage. Furthermore, it plays right into the hands of those unmarried couples or individuals who say they need coitus for their happiness.

4. The "argument from proportionalism." The proponents of this line of thought admit that contraception is a "physical evil" because it takes apart what God has joined together in the order of creation. However, they say that when there is a conflict of values, a physical evil is not a moral evil if there is a proportionate reason for allowing it. In the case at hand, contraception is seen as permissible if in the long run it fosters the values of marital fidelity, human sexuality, and the permanence of the marriage itself.

However, this argument is defeated on the very grounds it seeks for its justification. While an individual couple may say that the practice of contraception has made things easier between them and thus fostered those values, the wider evidence is against it. Increased divorce, increased nonmarital sex, and a general debasing of human sexuality have been the dominant characteristics of an age marked by an almost universal acceptance and use of contraception. (This idea is developed further in the section "Ecology of Morality.") Furthermore, this argument is dangerously similar to the following one.

5. "The end justifies the means." This approach also accepts that contraception is contrary to the natural order of creation but justifies it on the grounds of marital happiness, solving population problems, etc. It is rather obvious that this ends-means argument can be used to "solve" any kind of problem and has already resulted in such historic landmarks as the killing of six million Jews by the Nazis, the My Lai massacre by William Calley and company, and the current killing of literally millions of unborn children. As a principle for making morally right decisions, it offers no help.

Thus, many couples have been faced with the historic Christian view that the practice of contraception is morally wrong and with the additional fact that the typical pro-contraceptive arguments fail to be intellectually satisfying. However, can anything other than the historic tradition, anything in the way of explanation be offered in support of the belief that *natural* family planning is the best not only from the point of view of health, esthetics, cost, etc., but also from the point of view of morality? Again, several approaches should be investigated.

1. "An unnatural separation of powers." This approach, which has been explored well and in depth by Mary Joyce, notes that the natural law concerning man derives from an essential unity in the human person. Because one reveals himself in his or her actions, this essential unity of the person carries forward into a unity of his actions, at least his conscious ones. It is contrary to the very unity of his nature as a human being to act contrary to this essential unity. For example, in the human action of communication, there is a basic unity between what is in the mind and the expression of it — whether the communication is through the spoken or written word or by a nod of the head. When a person speaks or writes what he judges to be true, then he has respected the unity of his human nature, the order of creation. On the other hand, lying violates this essential unity. "Lying is an internal separation of a communication from its power to express and generate judgments truthfully."[1]

Coital intercourse is another and very special form of communication. Just as one of the powers of intellectual communication is the ability to create a new idea in the listener, so also one of the powers inherent in the human action of coitus is the power to create a new person in the womb of the mother. Contraception violates this unity of the action of its powers. Thus, contraception is "an internal separation of an interpersonal action of coital union from the fully human generative power that is internally structured in this action by the unity of the person's being."[2]

The basic assumption of this approach is that it is not humanly right to violate the unity of the person and his actions. To someone who can see that lying is morally wrong because it violates a meant-to-be unity between the person's judgment and his freely chosen action of expressing it, this argument from the unity of the coital act and its powers can be helpful in understanding why that unity may not be deliberately and internally separated. The proponents of this view note that this does not exclude coitus during the infertile period, for in such acts there is no internal separation of the act from one of its powers. The acts of coitus are accepted in their totality whether they are, in accord with human nature, able to result in conception or not.

This approach is one example of an explanation from the point of view of "natural law." It should be noted that natural law when applied to man and woman does not refer to any sort of physically unbreakable law of nature, such as the "law" of gravity. Rather, it refers to the way in which men and women *should* act to be in harmony with their very *being* and with the design of the Creator. For example, a man is physically able to become roaring drunk, make his way home, and literally terrorize his wife into submitting to coitus with him. In this example, we would think that such a man had acted against the natural law (or order of creation) in three ways: by getting roaring drunk in the first place, by terrorizing his wife, and by forcing her to have coitus when it had absolutely nothing to do with marital love, tenderness, affection, or the desire to conceive a child.

2. "A renewal of the marriage covenant." This approach can be meaningful to those who see coitus as morally proper only within marriage because it begins by asking, "For this couple, Richard and Mary, what is the moral difference between having coitus before marriage and having coitus only after they have married?" Certainly, between the week before marriage and the week after marriage there has been little change at the level of emotional love or affection. Yet a great many people and the weight of the Jewish-Christian tradition have seen and continue to see coitus prior to marriage as morally inappropriate. The answer provided in this second approach is that coitus becomes morally appropriate only after marriage because it is meant to be a renewal of the marriage covenant, and a couple obviously cannot renew what has not already taken place. In an authentic religious marriage covenant, the couple pledged before God in a true risk of faith their commitment to each other; they promised to exercise caring love for each other until they would be parted by death; they told both God and the world that they were entering upon a sacred unity with each other, that their very lives would be interpenetrated by the other. Thus, the coital act is meant to be a symbol of that unity, that caring love, that risk of faith by which they took each other for better and for worse.

In this approach, there is an emphasis on the risk inherent in pledging such life-long love and faithfulness to each other. Marital love, as contrasted with romantic or erotic love, means the loving acceptance of the other as he or she is now and will become during their life together. If one of the couple is naturally sterile, the faith risk of the marriage covenant does not allow the use of a substitute partner for childbearing purposes, nor does it allow divorce in order to have another marriage fruitful with children. In a similar manner, the faith risk entails the acceptance of that person's fertility as well. To practice contraception would be the equivalent of saying, "I accept you as represented by your body — but not your fertility." Thus, contraception goes contrary to the basic unity of the person and to the meaning of the coital act as a renewal of the love and faith risk of the original marriage covenant.

3. "What God has joined together . . . " This approach combines elements of each of the first two approaches. It notes first of all that there is rather obviously a natural unity arranged by the Creator in the coital act:—the development of marital love and affection and the procreation of children. It further notes that in this order of creation there is a rhythmic fertility cycle so that at some times the woman is fertile and at others she is not.

This approach then points to the fact that the coital act is rightly called the marriage act. The functions of developing marital love and procreating children are the traditional purposes of marriage, and the *combination* can be sought only through the coital act. Obviously, there are many ways of pursuing the development of marital love and affection, but there is only one way within the natural order of creation for pursuing the procreation of children. In the light of what was said in the preceding section, it might be more appropriate to call coitus the marriage *renewal* or affirmation act.

Since it has this unique place within marriage, the words of Jesus about marriage itself are appropriately applied to marital coitus: "What God has joined together, let no man divide" (Mark 10:9).

Now, rather obviously, the whole purpose of contraception is to divide what God has joined together in the coital act. As such, its function is to separate by positive interference the natural unity of sexual affection and procreation; it must be judged to be dividing what God has put together in a sacred unity and to be therefore contrary to God's design for human sexuality, love, and marriage. Natural family planning, on the other hand, respects what God has joined together and also what God himself has separated.

Anyone who finds this approach helpful may expect the skeptic to ask, "Well, why shouldn't we take apart what God has joined together?" Those who are oriented toward the natural might reply in a way something like this: "We don't know precisely why, but we have ample evidence that the ecological crises have resulted from man's refusing to respect the order within nature. We aren't saying that you can't use trees to build houses or put dams or bridges across rivers, etc., but we are saying that we have learned that it is to man's own interest to respect and to try to foster the natural order of things. The old idea that man can do anything he wanted to nature is truly obsolete."

Those who would answer the question of the skeptic from a religious point of view might answer in a way similar to this: "We honestly don't know all the reasons why we shouldn't divide what God has put together, whether we are talking about marriage itself or the coital marriage act. We can point to all sorts of tragedies that happen when a society starts to think it can take marriages apart at will—broken homes, increasing failure to really love and sacrifice in order to build the marriage, rising divorce rates, unstable homes and children, etc. We can also point to various unfortunate consequences of the practice and mentality of contraception. But in the last analysis, we have to admit that God didn't give us a book of proofs but rather asked for our faithful response to His word. We also believe that whether we are talking about the whole marriage relationship or the coital act, we are talking about very special human realities that are blessed by God. Because they are uniquely human and interpersonal and because they are sacred realities and far more than just a convenient social form or a biological unity, we have no right to take apart what God has put together."

Needless to say, the description of all of these approaches has been very incomplete. However, the surface has been scratched enough so that an open-minded reader can at least begin to see why many people remain quite unpersuaded by the arguments on behalf of contraception and what sort of moral reasoning is used to support the *natural*-family-planning-only view about birth regulation.

Moral considerations are persuasive only to those who already hold certain values and are frequently rejected by those who hold conflicting values. The couple who have elevated the idea that "sex is only (or mostly) for fun" to the place of their dominant value regarding sexuality may have considerable difficulty in becoming sensitive to the preceding considerations. However, we think that such couples are not the majority. Certainly, marital sex—in all its meaning, not just coitus—can be fun, but indications have appeared in the news media as well as in personal contacts that great numbers of people both young and old are searching for deeper meanings. To ask for such deeper meanings is to inquire ultimately how God meant His creature man to experience sexuality; it is the inquiry into the divine order of creation.

The Ecology of Morality

An inquiry into the order of creation regarding human sexuality, love, and marriage is in some ways similar to the inquiry into the balance of nature that we call ecology. We know that in the physical world one upset in nature leads to others, but what about in the world of human morality? Is there not a reality that we may call the ecology of morality (or an ecological morality)? What happens when one part of an overall sexual ethic is abandoned or rejected? Does that lead to an upset in other parts of the sexual ethic? Specifically, if the practice of contraception is contrary to the order of creation, will its acceptance as permissible lead to the acceptance of other actions that have been traditionally rejected as contrary to God's order of creation? In point of fact, the acceptance and rising use of contraception since the turn of the century (condoms became available in the mid nineteenth century after the discovery of vulcanizing rubber in 1843) has been followed by rising divorce rates, wife-swapping, increased frequency of nonmarital sex, and, most recently, huge increases in the number of abortions.

The question that thinking people simply *must* ask themselves is whether the rise in the use and acceptance of contraception as morally permissible and the rise in these other behaviors has been merely a historical coincidence or whether contraception has been a significant contributory cause to these other areas of sexual behavior.

This question is by no means new. Walter Lippmann, writing in 1929 and reflecting upon the sexual behavior of the 1920's, blamed the rise of sexual promiscuity squarely on the availability, acceptance, and use of contraceptives.[3] Lippman also criticized the idea of companionate, childless, trial "marriages," which were being proposed as a real advance made possible by the contraceptive separation of coitus and family raising. Such ideas strike us as terribly current, a product of the late 1960s and early 1970s, but they were being publicly promoted in the 1920s as well. In other words, proponents of companionate and temporary marriages were saying that contraception enabled them to promote new and radically changed ideas about human sexuality, love, and marriage.

Shortly after Lippmann's rather serious book appeared, Aldous Huxley published his short novel *Brave New World*,[4] which is still being reprinted and read today. Readers of that novel soon realize that the whole society of *Brave New World* is built upon the technology of sex. Contraception has almost completely divided coitus from procreation. Any contraceptive "mistakes" are taken care of at the abortion clinic. Just as logically in this novel, procreation (or rather the reproduction) of children is done by technology: test tube fertilization and development in bottles (artificial wombs) for nine months. Huxley carried the idea of companionate, temporary marriages one step further. Since the reproduction of children was all handled by technology and since the education of these children was in the hands of the state's full-care centers, there was no family and thus no need for parents. Thus, there was no marriage, and everybody was to belong sexually to everyone else. One is hard pressed to say whether Huxley was, at the time he wrote it in 1931, poking fun at the "new sexuality" that had come out of the 1920s or whether he was trying to crystal-ball the future. At any rate, today he looks in many ways, though not completely of course, very much like a "future-teller." It is common knowledge that some people seriously advocate letting the abortion clinic take care of contraceptive failures; others look forward to the day when technological reproduction is as efficient and as well accepted as is technological, contraceptive interference with procreation today.

Thus, we have seen writers of the 1920s and early 1930s spell out what they saw as the sexual logic of contraception. But what about the sexual theorists of today? Do they see any connection between contraception and other modes of sexual behavior? Would it not be a conclusive argument in favor of the idea of an "ecological morality of sex" if proponents of contraception themselves showed the connection between the acceptance of contraception and other forms of sexual or abortive behavior?

One prolific writer and advocate of contraception notes that "the contraceptive pill technology of the past twenty-five years has forced us to accept procreation and sexual intercourse as two distinct human actions, each governed by its own moral principles."[5] Taking for granted the use of our "sophisticated reproductive contraceptive technology," the author then describes some twenty possibilities for various sexual relationships, only one of which is permanent, monogamous marriage—which he thinks only a minority of people in the future will accept. The other nineteen include almost every imaginable combination: trial or two-step marriages, three-party marriages, polygamy for senior citizens, group marriages, temporary contractual marriages, stable unmarried cohabitation and unisex marriages. "Since we can no longer restrict sexual relations to a procreative function, homosexuality can no longer be condemned as immoral or unnatural merely because it is noncreative."[6] We would disagree with the author's conviction that the contraceptive technology has forced us to accept procreation and sexual intercourse as two distinct human actions, but we think that he offers an excellent example of the sexual logic of one who does accept that technological separation.

Michael Valente calls his book *Sex: The Radical View of a Catholic Theologian*, though it is in no way compatible with the official teaching of that church. Joining with those who rejected the official affirmation of the doctrine of noncontraception, and calling himself and other dissenters "revisionists," Valente states that "to accept the revisionist position of the liceity [moral lawfulness] of contraceptive use in marriage is not merely to find an exception to the natural law doctrine, but to destroy it."[7] He also questions the logic of those who would accept marital contraception but prohibit premarital or extramarital coitus.[8] Lest one think that such activity might be forbidden on the basis of Biblical statements, the author assures us that moral statements in the Bible simply reflect the writers' personal ideas about solving problems of living in accord with the dictates of the Judeo-Christian ethic. As isolated statements, they may be wrong and are therefore not binding.[9] Such reasoning, of course, puts Professor Valente out of touch not only with the Catholic tradition but with a great part of Protestant tradition as well.

However, he has now cleared the way to handle various sexual activities, some of which are rather specifically and vigorously opposed in the Bible. Thus,

"it seems unreasonable to maintain that there is a difference between allowing a husband and wife to use the condom and allowing them to have anal intercourse, since neither fulfills the natural law doctrine's requirement of insemination in the vagina. Likewise, there is no difference between using the condom and coitus interruptus or any of the other so-called sins prohibited under the doctrine, such as masturbation, homosexuality, and bestiality" [intercourse with an animal].

It would be hard to find a more explicit statement of the conviction by an advocate of contraception that the acceptance of marital contraception logically carries with it the acceptance of every imaginable sexual activity, provided such activity would not be condemned on other grounds, i.e., assault (rape), or the development of a bad self-image (promiscuity).

Shulamith Firestone is interested in a revolution between men and women that will include the abolition of the family as we now know it. Her interest in the question of contraception is not from the point of view of a moralist. Rather, Ms. Firestone looks forward to the dissolution of the family and sees technological contraception and reproduction as a necessary means for a revolutionary phaseout of the family. She argues that because of a combination of efficient contraception and nonfamily means of child rearing, it is possible for the first time to attack the family on the grounds that it is neither necessary nor the most efficient means of reproduction.[11] Aldous Huxley may have been either spoofing or ridiculing the sexual tendencies of Western civilization when he wrote *Brave New World*, but Ms. Firestone is perfectly serious in her advocacy of contraception and its societal consequences. In the system that she envisions, a woman's reproductive ability is a tyrant and women are to be freed from it by any and all possible means.[12] Furthermore, in her brave new world of efficient contraception, women and children should have and will have the freedom to do whatever they feel like doing sexually because there simply won't be any reason to refrain from gratification of their various urges.[13] Thus, once again, the cornerstone to both a philosophy and its implementation in eliminating marriage and the family has been technological contraception and its logical counterpart, technological reproduction.

We know that many people do not share the view that there is anything morally objectionable about contraception in marriage, even many people who are interested in natural family planning. We also think that contraception has become so much a part of "the American way of life" that many people have never given it much thought. Various circumstances have combined to make it a professional responsibility for us to read what others are saying and writing about sex, love, and marriage. Their writings have made us aware that there are certainly problems in modern marriage, many challenges to authentic love, and perhaps even increased difficulties in reaching sexual maturity. However, we cannot see that the "new directions" laid out for us by some of these writers lead anyplace except into a blind alley. We must ask our readers: Do you regard the abolition of marriage and the family as a real solution to the problems of the modern family? Do you regard the acceptance of any mutually agreeable sexual activity, even bestiality, as truly ennobling to man—or as consistent with your religion, whatever it may be?

Now, if those who are willing to spell out their theories and follow them to their logical conclusions tell us that to intellectually accept contraception is to logically accept anything and everything in the way of consenting sexual behavior, do we not have an excellent example of interlocking relationships, in other words, an ecology of morality? And when theories of sex end with such morally disastrous conclusions as these after starting with the acceptance of marital contraception, can those be criticized who hold that the starting point must be equally erroneous?

Much to the contrary, natural family planning is associated with a philosophy of sex, love, and marriage that sees the permanent marriage relationship as part of God's order of creation. It accepts the very real differences between man and woman. It does not magnify them but works with them to help the building of a sound and loving marriage relationship.

Certainly, the preceding analysis of the thought of some advocates of contraception has been brief and necessarily incomplete. However, we think that anyone who reads the books from which we have quoted will find that we have not distorted the authors' conclusions. We think it serves a useful purpose in the overall debate about the morality of contraception.

It has been suggested that those who see marital contraception as morally unacceptable do so out of a rather unthinking obedience to various religious authorities. We would hope that the preceding analyses would help to make it clear that at least some people who reject contraception on moral grounds do so because they have reviewed the philosophy, arguments, and conclusions of those who advocate marital contraception and have found them intellectually inadequate. Such people can only conclude that those who accept marital contraception as morally valid either (1) have a different set of standards about the whole ecology of sex, (2) have done so for reasons that are much less than intellectually satisfying, or (3) have done so simply out of a faith in various religious spokesmen who said that they saw nothing wrong with it. With regard to this latter point, many people would want to make a distinction between believing on the basis of a Biblical statement that they should not take apart what God has put together and believing on the basis of statements of various men that it didn't make any difference.

Theologically trained readers may complain that we have built a case by quoting only "far-out" writers rather than the more "moderate" advocates of contraception. Our response is simply that we have quoted those who have made a point of carrying the logic of technological, contraceptive birth control to its conclusions. The contraceptionists who sound more moderate either ignore these conclusions or brush them off with such statements as "We certainly don't intend *that*" or "*Those* things are contrary to the dignity of man." However, what counts is not their intention to stop at contraception but the underlying premises and the logical conclusions. Some of the same people who condemn the conclusions of Valente as being contrary to the dignity of man likewise criticize those who say that contraception is contrary to the dignity of man. They insist that the non-contraceptionists "prove" their conviction but have offered nothing by way of proof that they can logically accept contraception and yet condemn such activities as anal intercourse, etc. Considering contemporary sexual behavior, the burden of proof is certainly upon those who would say that the conclusions of Valente and company are not theoretically implicit in the acceptance of contraception.

Earlier we asked if it would not be a conclusive argument in favor of the idea of an "ecological morality of sex" if proponents of contraception themselves showed the connection between the acceptance of contraception and other forms of sexual behavior or abortive behaviors. We think that such proponents have done a good job of showing their conclusions about other forms of sexual behavior. But what about that "abortive behavior"? Is there any connection spelled out here?

I suggest to you that for the individual, the role of abortion will be, as it has been, the second line of defense against harmful pregnancy and the unwanted child. These are contraceptive failures. The societal role will require that we see family planning in a true light; no matter how thin you slice it, ladies and gentlemen, family planning is a euphemism. We don't intend or desire to prevent conception for conception's sake; we want to prevent conception because of what follows conception. Family planning is the prevention of births, and as birth is the end of a sequence which begins with the sexual urge, then family planning is anti-conception, anti-nidation, and the termination of the conceptus if implanted. This is the social role of abortion in the future.

The speaker was Professor Irwin Cushner of Johns Hopkins School of Medicine, addressing the Symposium on Implementation of Therapeutic Abortion held in Los Angeles in January 1971. He is quoted in *The Death Peddlers* by Paul Marx, in a chapter titled "How Abortionists Really Think."[14] In the thirty-three pages of this chapter, it is made abundantly clear that the scope of contraceptive family planning has now been widened to include postconception "family planning," that is, abortion at all stages. Thus, in this country the name of the Planned Parenthood Association and that of its late president, Dr. Alan Guttmacher, have become almost synonymous with the efforts to gain public acceptance for abortion as just one more means of family planning. People who want to see the planning of the abortionists to get tax money, to deceive women into thinking that they are just "menstruating" when they are really aborting, and to generally increase the abortion business should read this little book by Professor Marx. When these indications are coupled to the statement of the Presbyterian Report[15] that accepted abortion as a backstop to contraception, we find it hard to deny a very real link between the two. We do not know how people can avoid the conclusion that the widespread acceptance of contraception has been responsible for the acceptance of abortion. Thus, there is one more example of the "ecology of sexual morality."

In summary, we have found no indications that the acceptance, use, and philosophy of contraception have led to the raising of public and personal sexual morality since the turn of the century and especially in the forty-odd years since it was first given some religious acceptance. On the contrary, we think that history has shown that Walter Lippman in 1929 was quite perceptive when he linked the use of contraception with other forms of sexual behavior he regarded as immoral.

If this perception is correct, then there is obviously much more at stake in the natural family planning movement than just helping people to learn about the various signs of fertility and ovulation. History would suggest that when a civilization as a whole abandons a sexual ethic that is truly uplifting and in accord with what is best in man and woman and replaces it with an ethic that cannot really say no to anything mutually pleasurable, then that civilization cannot long endure. Such a thought suggests that the acceptance, use, and philosophy of natural family planning may be a positive and constructive element not only at the level of the individual marriage but also at the larger level of society.

References

[1]Mary Joyce, *The Meaning of Contraception* (Staten Island, New York: Alba House, 1970), p. 26.

[2]Ibid., p. 8.

[3]Walter Lippmann, *A Preface to Morals* (New York: The Macmillan Company, 1929).

[4]Aldous Huxley, *Brave New World* (New York: Harper & Row, 1969; first published in 1932).

[5]Robert T. Francoeur, *Eve's New Rib: Twenty Faces of Sex, Marriage and Family* (New York: Harcourt, Brace, Jovanovich, 1972, p. 4.

[6]Ibid., p. 223.

[7]Michael F. Valente, *Sex: The Radical View of a Catholic Theologian* (New York: Bruce, 1970), p. 126.

[8]Ibid.

[9]Ibid., p. 147.

[10]Ibid., p. 126.

[11]Shulamith Firestone, *The Dialectic of Sex: The Case for Feminist Revolution* (New York: William Morrow and Company, Inc. 1970), p. 250.

[12]Ibid., p. 233.

[13]Ibid., p. 236.

[14]Paul Marx, *The Death Peddlers,* Collegeville, Minn. (St. John's University Press, 1971), p. 122.

[15]Previously referred to in Chapter 2, reference 1. See also Chapter 2, reference 4.

Notes

Notes

9

Marriage Building with Natural Family Planning

Marriage Building

When the Couple to Couple League was first started, it was not its intention to get involved in the rather huge challenge of trying to help married couples improve their marriages. Practically a whole industry of psychiatrists, psychologists, clergy, marriage counselors, and organizations was already working at this task. Thus, CCL had and continues to have as its main objective the more limited purpose of helping couples to learn how to practice natural family planning. However, right from the beginning it was realized that a couple who wanted to practice natural family planning successfully had to have certain attitudes. The old idea of the wife being there in bed as the immediate relief valve for any and all sexual urges of her husband had to be replaced by something more meaningful without denying that the relief of sexual tension can be a valid reason for marital coitus.

As a result, two things happened. First of all, leader couples at CCL meetings have talked briefly about the necessity of marital teamwork, mutual decision making, open communication, and the importance of expressing marital love and affection in nongenital ways. The second thing that happened is that various couples have told Couple to Couple League leader couples such things as "CCL has saved our marriage," "Our marriage has become richer as a result of CCL," etc. Of course, CCL has not really saved any marriages; the couples themselves, with the help of God, have healed or saved their own marriages by changing their marital attitudes and behavior.

At any rate, whatever the limited purpose of CCL as an organization, the experience of people associated with it has been that the practice of natural family planning has frequently had the value of helping to improve shaky marriages and to make good ones even better. However, such marriage building doesn't just happen, nor has it been the result of going to a CCL series for a course on having a happy marriage. Rather it

179

has been the result of pursuing other values that are all part of the "logic" involved in natural family planning.

Mutual Decision Making

Natural family planning is built upon mutual fertility awareness and decision making. During each menstrual cycle, the couple become aware of the changes in the wife's fertility pattern. We don't attempt to lay down any hard-and-fast rules about how *both* husband and wife are involved in this, but the following guidelines have been derived from the successful practice of various couples.

1. The process of fertility awareness should not be left up to the wife alone. There are several things that will normally be done by the wife, such as taking mucus observations, but there are other things that can and should be done by the husband.

2. The husband should be involved in some of the daily practice of fertility awareness. Obviously, if he is traveling or has to leave the house hours before his wife gets up, modifications will have to be made; however, under normal conditions he should participate. For example, among many couples who use the sympto-thermal method, it is the practice for the husband to give his wife the thermometer in the morning and to record the temperatures.

3. Decision making should be mutual. The husband should be actively engaged in the interpretation of the signs of fertility. Some couples think that the decision to resume coitus should be *only* the husband's, thus forcing him to become involved in the art of interpretation. These people want to do everything possible to avoid the situation where the husband leaves everything up to the wife and places her under a certain psychological pressure to announce "safe day" as quickly as possible. If the only possible way to overcome such an attitude is to leave the decision making entirely to the husband, then we would have to go along with it reluctantly. Such a couple would have a problem that has nothing to do with natural family planning but was merely brought to the surface by the occasion of having to work together. Once on the surface, it can be dealt with constructively. It would be something entirely different if the couple agreed that the husband should make the final and important decisions because of his role as "head of the family." However, we think that normally it should be a matter of mutual interpretation and decision making.

All of this should not give the impression that there is some huge and difficult decision to make every month. Normally speaking, the rules of natural family planning make the wife's fertility stage rather self-evident, but even an easily made decision is still a decision. When the interpretation of the signs of fertility is difficult for an inexperienced couple, they may decide to seek help from others who are more experienced. Providing such counsel is another service of the Couple to Couple League and other natural family planning groups.

Recurring Thought about Meaning

Another way in which the commitment to natural family planning contributes to marriage building is that it provides the couple with a regularly recurring opportunity to think about the meaning of their marriage, sex, and their spiritual values. This is nothing new in human sexuality. As mentioned earlier, for over three thousand years the Orthodox Jew has been required by his Law to refrain from sexual relations at certain times. Through the observance of the Law, the believer was thus asked to think about God, the ultimate lawgiver, and to reaffirm his spiritual values.

Many Christians believe in a reality called "the communion of saints" in the creed. One aspect of this belief might be called the spiritual unity of mankind. The prayers, good deeds, and sacrifices of one person can help someone else through the universal mediation of Christ. Why is this mentioned here? Many people who are interested in natural family planning are also concerned about the degenerating sexual morality that characterizes a significant part of our society. The mere fact that a couple make a commitment to natural family planning does not mean that they are never going to experience any difficulties of self-control during the time when they have decided not to have coitus. For one who believes in this spiritual unity of mankind, such difficulties can be spiritualized; they can be transformed into a positive work for the up-lifting of the sexual habits of the world in general or of other particular persons in the world, their children, for example. The Christian couple can go even further and unite any of their difficulties with the sacrifice of Christ in a living prayer for divine guidance and the grace to be good parents. Such a positive approach can bring the couple closer together at the spiritual level and be a most effective marriage builder.

A Remedy for Satiety

When the popular television show "All in the Family" dealt with wife-swapping (October 28, 1972), the topic of sexual satiety was touched upon indirectly. The wife-swapping couple explained that they had taken up this way of life because the zip had gone out of their own married life. That was about as close as anyone could get on television to saying, "We became tired of each other as sex partners, we've had so much of each other, we're bored." We have seen no studies that have analyzed the wife-swapping scene, but we find it hard to imagine that couples who had solid and satisfying marriages would be very interested in such activity. We would be willing to guess that the couple in the television show gave a fairly good reason why some couples take that route in an effort to do something about a crumbling relationship. Interestingly enough, wife-swapping was infrequently practiced before the Pill gave people an added feeling of security. Is it merely coincidental that the growth of wife-swapping and the use of the Pill occurred at the same time? Could it be that the practice of contraception has increased the quantity but lowered the quality of marital coitus? It would seem that the quantitative approach to sex easily results in "having it more but enjoying it less."

Periodic abstinence is good for the marriage relationship because it helps avoid the feeling of sexual satiation, the feeling of having too much quantity, and a corresponding lack of joy and meaning. Such voluntary and mutual refraining from intercourse is part of the normal pattern of natural family planning and as such can contribute to building the marriage. Once the couple resume intercourse it is a common experience for them to have a heightened appreciation of it. This has led to the saying among some couples who practice natural family planning, "Every cycle has a period of courtship followed by a honeymoon."

Nongenital Ways of Marital Affection

As indicated above, when a husband and wife are in a period of refraining from coitus, they do not simply forget or ignore each other. Rather, it can be compared with the period of courtship that preceded the marriage and honeymoon. There are very significant differences between a chaste and loving premarital courtship and the regular "courtship" phrase of natural family planning, for the married couple may morally engage in nongenital behavior that would be highly inappropriate for the unmarried. However, the comparison we would want to make still has validity. During the period before marriage, the couple with a commitment to premarital purity looked for and found nongenital and nonpassionate ways of expressing their love and affection. The fact that they did not have intercourse provided no deterrent to their love; on the contrary, the other little niceties of courtship helped to develop their relationship. Tenderness and gentleness instead of passion, conversation rather than coitus, helped to broaden and deepen their friendship.

In a similar fashion, when a married couple choose to refrain from intercourse for a period of time — whatever the reason — they should remember some of the pleasantries of courtship. Conversation without coitus is once again especially appropriate. Her making him a special dinner or his taking her out to dinner provide traditional ways of courtship for the married as well as the unmarried. His performance of some of the household jobs that she has wanted done or his taking out the garbage without complaint can be most helpful in the process of marital courtship. So also can be her verbal thanks for such little things and her compliments for his help with the children. Some couples find that a bit of cuddling is very helpful; the wife feels more loved for her own sake when her husband puts his arm around her and sprinkles their conversation with a few kisses without coitus than when it is known that all such activity is simply a preliminary to coital gratification. There is no universal recipe for the periodic courtship-without-coitus phase of marriage; an excellent exercise in marital communication would be a discussion of what each might do for the other in such periods. The important thing is that they still show each other that they care and are friends. In this way, they can actively work against one of the worst enemies of the marital relationship — taking each other for granted.

Increased Respect

If the feeling of being taken for granted is a prime cause of marital discontent, the feeling of being used must run a close second. For reasons that are probably obvious to most readers, this is particularly true of women. When the frequency and the conditions of intercourse lead a woman to feel that she is being used pretty much just as a means of sexual relief for her husband, her respect for him is hardly increased, no matter how sympathetic she is to his sexual urges. On the other hand, when couples give up their practice of contraception and turn to natural family planning, it is a fairly common experience for the wife to develop greater respect for her husband.

Encountering Difficulties

Even with firm moral convictions that natural family planning is the only way to go, even with convictions that the natural way is not only best for the individual couple but even for our civilization, couples will still experience occasional difficulties. Natural family planning involves some voluntary sexual self-restraint, and that can be difficult. Some experienced couples may refrain from genital contact for less than a week; others go for two or three weeks or longer without genital relations. The approach taken to any difficulties will have much to do with the couple's happiness and success.

We certainly don't have a ready-made formula that we can hand to

184

every couple that guarantees they will have no problems. However, common sense plus the experience of couples practicing natural family planning suggest some thoughts and guidelines that may be helpful not just in developing a positive approach to difficulties but also in developing a deeper, more mature marriage relationship. Indeed, it is a frequent comment from couples we meet in CCL that natural family planning demands a certain amount of maturity to begin with but results in an even more mature, stable, and happy marital relationship. Repeatedly, we have been told by others that the efforts involved in natural family planning have been repaid tenfold in marriage enrichment.

Accept Difficulties as an Enriching Part of Life

The famous Jewish psychiatrist Victor Frankl reflected deeply upon his experiences as a prisoner in the Nazi concentration camps during World War II. His book *Man's Search for Meaning* is the type that you can hardly put down, and many read it at one sitting. (A common experience is that it quickly makes the rounds in a neighborhood because it is something people want to share.) He notes that

suffering is an ineradicable part of life, even as fate and death. Without suffering and death human life cannot be complete. The way in which a man accepts his fate and all the suffering it entails, the way in which he takes up his cross, gives him ample opportunity — even under the most difficult circumstances — to add a deeper meaning to his life . . . . Everywhere man is confronted with fate, with the chance of achieving something through his own suffering. [1]

Of course, whatever difficulties one may encounter in natural family planning are different from the sufferings Frankl and his associates endured in prison, not just because the natural family planning difficulties are much, much less severe but also because these lesser problems are freely accepted as part of the price of pursuing and upholding certain values.

Another indication that the willing acceptance of difficulties can be a real source of meaning and life-enrichment is the statement of Jesus: "Whoever tries to gain his own life will lose it; whoever loses his life for my sake will gain it" (Matthew 10:39). That doesn't apply just to ultimate martyrdom; it also applies to the little martyrdoms of everyday life in which we "die" to some expression of self-will and find ourselves correspondingly enriched, especially if we have done it for the sake of Christ. Many of the "Jesus people" witness to the fact that by giving up their free-love sexual activity for Christ, they have indeed become more free and more loving as total persons.

Count Your Blessings

One of the most unfortunate things that can occur in any person's life is the state of feeling sorry for oneself. It is quite imaginable that occasionally men and women, whether married or single, may start to feel sorry for themselves because they think they are not having as much sexual pleasure and fun as other people. (And that "as much" can mean either quantity or quality.) For the single, such thoughts, if allowed to develop, can dispose them to engage in fornication; for the married, we would imagine that such attitudes weaken their defenses to the temptation to engage in various forms of adultery.

It is hard to imagine that some men and women practicing natural family planning have not also been tempted to feel sorry for themselves during times of genital continence. Such people may choose to reject such temptations by reflecting on their blessings. Or, to look at the other side of the coin, they can realize how much worse it could be. In any marriage, one of the couple could have an injury, an infection, or some other problem that would mean having no coital relations for a long time — months, or even for life. And how much better to go to bed at night with a faithful and loving spouse than to go to bed alone, wondering where your spouse is.

More positively, married couples should be glad they are not endangering each other's health or taking the life of a newly conceived child through the current popular forms of birth control. They can be proud of the fact that they have learned to understand this aspect of human nature; millions of people wouldn't know where to start. We think it is a fundamental rule of life: Count your blessings.

Take One Day at a Time

Another attitude that is helpful in dealing with any sexual frustration that may arise is "Let each day take care of itself." We are married for life, but we only have to live one day at a time. In the Lord's Prayer, we pray only for this day's bread.

Keep Communication Open

Throughout the whole range of the experience of marriage, open communication is a necessity. Many little problems can be solved or greatly reduced simply by talking about them, sometimes just by admitting they are there. If, for example, the husband should be feeling a few urges, knows he must exercise self-retraint, but is having a bit of difficulty, the situation may be greatly relieved by his telling his wife the situation. It will probably be much more helpful if they are both willing to joke about it: "Honey, I'm feeling oversexed . . ." A couple who can laugh together at any of the difficulties of sexual restraint are on the road to sexual maturity and are miles ahead of the couple who begin to feel sorry for themselves.

Use Common Sense and Mutual Support

An attitude of mutual care and support is important. Part of this is by way of communication but also included are some little things. For example, if a husband has told his wife, "When you wear that shorty nightgown, all I can think of is making love to you all the way," then it is simply a matter of common sense for her not to tease his imagination in that way when they have already chosen to refrain from coitus at that time.

In a similar vein, common sense dictates that they should avoid TV shows, movies, magazines, and books that have a definitely erotic effect. Many people have a sexual drive that receives ample stimulation just from being alive and in the presence of one's spouse. Why complicate matters by patronizing those whose sales effort is directed toward further sexual stimulation?

Furthermore, it is common experience that alcoholic beverages can reduce inhibitions, make one feel sexier, and generally create problems with self-restraint. Again, it is simply a matter of common sense not to make things harder for oneself by drinking to the point where these things occur. For some, that may mean complete abstinence from alcohol; for others, it may mean stopping after one drink. People who take two or more drinks are quite probably creating unnecessary difficulties for themselves and their spouses.

In a similar vein, Dr. Pierre E. Slightam has suggested that a healthy diet makes it easier to practice natural family planning. "Many women would have more regularly spaced, natural periods and menstrual cycles if they would eat better."[2] Dr. Slightam counsels his patients to avoid as far as possible the "factory foods" from which the nutritional value has been taken, e.g., white flour and sugar, to avoid or limit the intake of caffeine, and to eat natural foods. He believes that a one-a-day type vitamin supplement may be helpful to make up for the deficiencies in today's processed foods. This applies to men as well as women, because an improper diet results in poor body balance and may provide increased difficulties with one's nervous system and self-control.

Don't Blame the Natural Family Planning Decision for Basic Marital Problems

This warning is addressed primarily to those who feel that the decision not to practice contraception was more or less imposed on them from the outside. Thus, it becomes a convenient scapegoat for all sorts of problems, especially by those who would see more coital relations as the answer to their marital needs.

Dr. Max Levin, a Jewish neurologist and clinical professor at the New York Medical College, some time ago addressed an audience that was acquainted with the outlook of some Catholics on this matter:

> In cases where rhythm is a problem, the husband regards sex not as something he can give his wife but as something to give *himself* as a compensation for his various grievances. In cases I have seen where periodic continence was presented as an intolerable burden, there has not been a single case where I didn't find something seriously wrong with the marriage. There was no love, no spirit of devotion. One or both partners were immature, egocentric, selfish. They were wrapped up in themselves, not each other. It was not the frustration of the rhythm method that was disturbing them. Even if the Church were to change the rules and raise all bars, they would still be miserable living together. What they need is not permission to use other contraceptive methods. They need therapy.[3]

Make the Decision Your Own

When a policy of marital noncontraception is also the official teaching of major religious bodies—Roman Catholicism, the Eastern Orthodox churches, Orthodox Judaism—then it is quite possible that certain believers will accept the teaching in faith but in a most grudging way. Their attitude may be that this is something imposed upon them by some old-fogey ecclesiastics, and consequently the practice of periodic marital continence may seem like quite a burden indeed. Now, however meritorious it may be for such people to accept what they feel is a burden out of a spirit of loyalty and faith, their own religious leaders would greatly prefer that they internalize this decision, that they make the decision on the basis of a moral conviction that the practice of contraception fails to uphold the divine order of creation and the sacredness of human sexuality.

Such couples might do well to remember that other couples are making the same decision for reasons that have nothing to do with religious faith; we would hope that both types of couples will find in these discussions various facts and reasons that will clarify and support their decision.

Expand Your Ideas About Making Love

You have probably noticed that we have regularly used the technical terms "coitus" or "genital relations" as substitutes for the less technical terms "sexual intercourse" and "sexual relations" and have generally avoided the term "making love." Our reason for doing this has been very deliberate. Our culture has tended to identify "sex" with "genitals," "sexual intercourse" with "genital intercourse," and "making love" with "genital intercourse." In reality, any sort of human interchange between any man and any woman can be termed an intercourse that is sexual in a broad sense of the term. However, because of the common limitation of the term "sexual intercourse" to coitus, we have followed the general usage in this manual.

When it comes to the term "making love," who can say that any particular act of coitus is one of "making" love? The term is used frequently for coitus outside of marriage, where the appropriate moral terms are "fornication," "adultery," and even "prostitution." Even within marriage, many honest couples will admit that there is no direct and necessary relationship between coitus and the "making" or "expression" of love. Sometimes, their marital coitus is very expressive of love and is truly constructive, or a "making" of marital love. At other times, their marital coitus is hardly more than a sexual relief mechanism. This is not to level some sort of condemnation of the idea of coitus for sexual relief, but it is to say that honesty requires that we admit that "making love" is frequently just a euphemism that is more useful in describing what coitus is meant to be at its best instead of what it actually is. Thus, we think that our talk about sex would be better off if we eliminated any sort of identity between "making love" and "coitus." On the other hand, we should use the term "making love" in a much wider context. There are all sorts of "love making" or "love building" activities that have nothing to do with coitus.

Just a few days before writing these lines a friend who knew we were working on the manual gave us a couple of short articles on marriage. One of them carried the following thoughts by an anonymous contributor.

Each couple will need to find or rediscover for themselves the ways to say, "I love you and I want you to be happy." It is an art that is not acquired without effort. It may include:

HIS remembering the good-bye kiss or the hello kiss.
HIS bringing her something occasionally (even a bag of peanuts) to let her know that he thought of her during the day.
HIS sharing the goals and problems of his work with her.
HIS doing at least the masculine jobs around the house.
HIS helping in the physical care and particularly the discipline of the children.
HER preparing his favorite meal even though it is by no means her favorite.
HER sprucing up before he is due home at night.

HER overcoming shyness to give a spontaneous and unexpected physical show of affection.

HER learning enough about it to appreciate his sports or political interests.

The project may be as subtle and as long-range as HER sensitizing him to the emotional element of love and HIS educating her in sensuality and the physical response.

Cultivating a sense of proportion and sense of humor . . . in all areas, but, particularly, concerning the sexual life. Laughter can relieve tension. *Love is not necessarily increased by solemnity.*

We would go even further and try to examine the "love-making" aspects of what typically takes place when a couple engage in the coital embrace. Typically, they begin with romantic talk and kissing, then engage in necking and petting, and all of this may have been done fully or partially clothed. Then, they engage in the coital act; soon the husband alone or husband and wife together experience orgasm, and rather shortly thereafter it is typically all over. Now, of all these elements, can we say definitely that some are more constructive of "love-making" than others? In other words, can we say for sure that in this typical series of marital activities the actual coitus and orgasm are any more constructive of the love relationship than what is typically called the foreplay? Or could a good case be made for the statement that the foreplay, the talk, and the kissing and petting are at least equally constructive of the marital love relationship?

We have heard from several sources that some Europeans, Orientals, and Americans think that the practice of coitus reservatus is the height of the art of love-making. (Coitus reservatus means engaging in physical coitus but controlling oneself so that neither party has orgasm.) Now, sperm may be present in the slight nonorgasmic lubricatory discharge that comes from the penis of the sexually stimulated man, and thus genital contact and certainly the practice of coitus reservatus are excluded on practical grounds during the fertile period. Furthermore, such a practice carries with it a certain risk of accidental orgasm, especially among those who are accustomed to orgasmic coitus. But still, one wonders whether these people may not have a grain of truth in their de-emphasis on orgasm and their positive emphasis on some of the other aspects of erotic marital love.

At any rate, marital continence is not the same thing as living as brother and sister; it is not the continence of those who have dedicated themselves to a single, celibate state. The periodic marital continence of natural family planning does exclude coitus and genital contact, but it does not exclude the sexual intimacy of kissing, necking, and petting. Certainly, it takes self-control to firmly hug and kiss one's spouse and not think immediately or exclusively in terms of carrying through to orgasm, but this type of self-control is part of what is meant by the development of sexual maturity.

Now, some couples may decide to engage in no more than a kiss goodbye, hello, and a quick good-night. They may find that to engage in any further intimacy puts too much strain on one or both parties. Other couples may find that they can engage in these marital pleasantries without feeling any sort of overpowering drive toward coitus; they may find that such activity helps reduce sexual tension. Most of these latter couples will have arrived at this state only little by little. We only wish to point out that sexual self-control within natural family planning does not necessarily mean avoiding all husband-and-wife contact that is sexually arousing. It also includes being able to experience moderate sexual stimulation and still being able to control oneself from going further. We would think that one of the best times to begin to develop this sort of self-control would be during the *infertile* times so that if passion should take over, the complete act of coitus and orgasm would not result in pregnancy.

Couples who manage to expand their ideas about making love will also be less concerned or anxious in looking forward to the resumption of coital relations when they find the indications of infertility. If coitus is simply one of many ways in which they have learned to express their marital love and affection, then the first day of the infertile phase will not take on undue importance. Perhaps they won't feel like engaging in coitus that night anyway.

Quite obviously, this process of expanding one's view of the practice of love-making deemphasizes the quantitative approach that has been so much a part of our culture especially since Dr. Kinsey reported on his study of the coital customs of married Americans—so many times per week for this age group and so many times for that group. In effect, the approach inherent in natural family planning says, "Dare to be different. Put more emphasis on the quality of your marital love as a whole than on the quantity of coital acts. Learn to be lovers." Another writer put it this way some years ago:

> If a husband and wife have not learned in a few years how to give themselves to each other totally in the intimacy of an understood look, they had better get busy learning how to love each other. They are simply lousy lovers. And I don't care if they hustle off to bed every night of the week for the so-called marital embrace. If that is the only love-making they do, they are at best only half-alive.[4]

Expand the Meaning of the Marital Embrace

Just as it is necessary to expand the meaning of love-making to include many noncoital activities, so also is it necessary to expand the meaning of the coital act. If it is seen only in terms of biological urges, it is being viewed too narrowly. We believe that it may be helpful to make use of some of the ideas touched upon earlier in order to have a more adequate understanding of the meaning of the coital embrace.

Marriage is both a state and a process of being. We have all heard talk about "the married state," which refers to the status of the couple before God and the world. For some reason, we have heard less talk about "the marriage process," which refers to how this man and wife are continuing to develop their marital status with each other. Perhaps one reason for this is that it is a relatively easy and one-time step to enter the married state, but the marriage process is never completed. To put it another way, when two people commit themselves in marriage, they promise to give of themselves in a caring love for each other for the rest of their lives. They give themselves without reservation to each other for better or for worse. However, most married people will acknowledge that it is easier to make this commitment than it is to engage in the day-by-day process of carrying it out and renewing it.

In this perspective, the coital embrace is seen as a unique expression of married love; it is seen as embodying and renewing in a symbolic way their original marriage commitment of *total* giving to each other. In this way, the meaning of the coital embrace takes on the very meaning of marriage itself; this is certainly a view of coitus that is considerably more expansive than the idea that coitus is chiefly the expression of biological urges.

In such an expanded view of the meaning of the coital embrace there is no room for contraception. The coital renewal of the marriage covenant calls to mind the couple's vow of giving *without* reservation to each other, but contraceptive coitus is very simply the expression of the sexual encounter *with* serious reservation. As such, it fails to fulfill the rich and real meaning of the marital embrace.

Be Positive About the Difference

Because couples who practice natural family planning are apparently a minority with respect to those who use mechanical and chemical contraceptives and abortifacients, they are frequently not only soft-spoken about their conviction but even apologetic. However, there are increasing reasons to be more positive. We have already reviewed such values as esthetics, health, cost, and life of the newly conceived baby, and we have spent time on religious and moral values that are involved in the choice of methods for birth regulation.

We have heard from various couples who made a thoughtful decision to use only natural family planning and who yet found themselves at a loss for words to answer the question, "Well, what difference does it make which way you choose? After all, we all have the same purpose in mind." We have already tried to provide a response to that at the level of moral principles in Chapter 8 but a related example may be helpful.

Periodically, we read about a "marriage contract" in which the couple agree to a five-year term of legal marriage with an option to renew; sometimes the "contract" is for no time period but lists the various conditions under which they will remain married or will call it quits. The aim is quite simple: to eliminate the risks of an unhappy marriage.

Most people contemplating Christian marriage likewise hope to avoid an unhappy marriage. If they have any idea of what marriage is, they realize it is a risk, so they try to cut down the risks. They try to find a mate who is truly compatible; they try to have some financial basis for living. Many will postpone the wedding until some milestone has been achieved, such as graduation, military discharge, or employment. But still, within the Christian principle, when that couple finally marries, they take each other for better or for worse. If the sky falls in on their plans a week after marriage, they are still married. They have accepted each other, committed themselves to each other in a risk of faith and love. The unconditional character of their commitment is the core of what makes their union a marriage.

Both the "five-year option" pair and the carefully selective couple hoped to avoid an unhappy marriage, and both took steps to reduce the risks. However, in the first case, they destroyed the very meaning of marriage, while in the second case they accepted it for all that it is.

Contraception is like the "five-year option." It so absolutizes the elimination of risk that it contradicts the meaning of the sexual act as a renewal of the marriage convenant for better or for worse. On the other hand, the couple who practice natural family planning may engage in the sexual embrace only when the possibility of conception has been naturally reduced or eliminated. When they engage in the marital embrace, they—unlike our second couple—accept it for all that it is, thereby keeping it as a symbol of unconditional giving of each to the other. The difference is significant.

Develop Authentic Notions About Freedom

A proper approach to freedom is helpful in natural family planning, and a false idea of freedom can bring chaos to a marriage. Some people don't want to marry because they feel it will restrict their sexual freedom, and others pursue freedom and happiness in extramarital affairs. Such unfortunate people are more slave than free.

If the coital embrace is viewed almost solely in terms of being the result of various biological or romatic urges, then it tends to be seen as "inevitable" or "absolutely necessary." Such a limited view about the meaning of the marital embrace leads to erroneous and narrow conclusions about our freedom to say "yes" or "no."

Most of us have found that freedom isn't really free. To be free to run a mile without stopping, we have to put forth a great deal of training effort. The same is true of sexual freedom. To be sexually free means to have enough sexual self-possession so that we are masters over our urges and can place sex at the service of authentic love. To attain that degree of freedom requires the help of God, and no one should feel ashamed at admitting his or her need for divine help in this area of life.

The Christian will recall the frequently quoted words of Jesus, "And the truth will make you free." Less frequently quoted is the preceding sentence, "If you continue in my word, you are truly my disciples and you will know the truth" (John 8:31-32). Thus, in the Christian perspective, authentic freedom comes from discipleship, and no one has ever said that authentic Christian discipleship was easy. Furthermore, the statement of Jesus that "without me you can do nothing" makes it a responsibility for those who wish to be his disciples to acknowledge their need for his help and to pray for the gift and development of authentic sexual freedom.

* * *

Current awareness teaches us that many people do not see everything the way we have written in this manual; many have never thought about some of the things we have touched upon. Though we have written many words on a number of related topics, this has not been the place to develop in any adequate way a complete rationale of natural family planning or a critique of the contraceptive and the abortacient approaches. Despite these limitations, we are led to believe from our correspondence that the preceding considerations may prove helpful to people who have already made the decision for natural family planning and to those who are still in the process of making up their minds.

194

Furthermore, we think that a great many couples of good-will have made a decision for contraception based on a seriously limited consideration of all the values involved; we would hope that many such couples will reevaluate that decision and choose to follow only the natural way in the future, and perhaps this book may offer them some food for thought. At any rate, we would hope that even our critics would agree that a well-rounded, consistent, and intellectually satisfying case can be made for the statement that natural family planning is the best approach to birth regulation because it is the only one that is at the same time—

—highly effective

—without medical hazards

—morally and religiously acceptable

—humanly challenging and appropriate

—and a marriage enriching process in which husbands and wives are considered as creatures of God, called and empowered to respond to the divine order of creation.

References

[1]Victor Frankl, *Man's Search for Meaning* (New York: Washington Square Press, Inc., 1963), pp. 106-107.

[2]Pierre E. Slightam, in *Coverline* (New Haven: Natural Family Planning Association) vol. 2, no. 16, Spring 1973.

[3]Max Levin, "Sexual Fulfillment with Rhythm," in *Marriage* (June, 1966), p. 32.

[4]Frank M. Wessling, "Is It Immature Loving?" in *America* (May 2, 1964), p. 595.

10

The Rules of Natural Family Planning

The following rules are intended to summarize much of what has been written in the preceding chapters, and they are intended to be understood in the light of those explanations. Some of the rules apply to everyone; others are for special situations. Be sure to see Section A in Chapter 6 for more complete guidelines.

Important Reminders

1. Keep loving each other regardless of whether you are having coitus or not. Periods of sexual restraint can be periods of care and consideration; they need not be periods of restraint from all physical embracing. Keep up the marital courtship and enjoy the honeymoon later on.

2. Keep your attitudes positive and work together as a team. With the proper attitudes you can go for extended periods without coitus, and your marriage will grow rather than weaken.

3. Keep good records on a daily basis. Sloppy records greatly complicate the process of interpretation.

4. Feel free to seek technical or personal support from members of the Couple to Couple League or other natural family planning groups.

Review of Terms

Phase I: Relatively infertile period.
Phase II: Fertile or possible fertile period.
Phase III: Postovulation, absolutely infertile period.
Pre-ovulation base: The level of the pre-ovulation temperatures established by the normal high temperatures in Phase I, especially by the six temperatures just prior to the beginning of the thermal shift.

Thermal shift: The postovulation rise in temperatures sustained in an overall rising or elevated pattern for at least three days, reaching and staying at a level usually .4 (4/10) of 1° F. above the pre-ovulation base.

Mucus-only method: A system of fertility awareness utilizing only the mucus symptom and not using the cervix and temperature signs of ovulation.

Sympto-thermal method: A system of fertility awareness that makes use of all the signs of ovulation—cervix, cervical mucus, and basal temperatures.

Temperature-only method: A system of fertility awareness utilizing only the basal temperatures.

21-day rule: A rule for establishing the length of the relatively infertile phase based on the shortest previously recorded cycle: Shortest Cycle - 21 days = Last Day of Phase I.

Avoiding Pregnancy During Phase I

Be aware of breakthrough bleeding and avoid any genital contact during bleeding or apparent menstruation that has not been preceded by a thermal shift in the previous cycle.

The most effective policy is to apply the 21-day rule. Do not have coitus on days past the last day of Phase I as indicated by the 21-day rule. If mucus appears before the last day indicated by the 21-day rule, consider that Phase II has begun and refrain from coitus.

A less effective policy but still relatively efficient for couples experienced in cervix and mucus signs would be:

1. Apply the 21-day rule. If mucus appears before the last day indicated by the 21-day rule, consider that Phase II has begun.

2. On days past the limits of the 21-day rule: (a) do not have coitus on consecutive days; (b) consider that Phase II has begun when mucus appears; and (c) once definitely in Phase II as established by the mucus and/or cervix signs, refrain from coitus until the beginning of Phase III as established by the sympto-thermal rules.

Avoiding Pregnancy During Phase II

Avoid all coitus and genital contact from the beginning of Phase II until the beginning of Phase III has been established by the sympto-thermal rules.

Sympto-thermal Rules for Establishing the Beginning of Phase III

1. *Perfect Coinciding (PC):* When all the signs coincide, Phase III begins on the evening of the day indicated by

(a) the third day of full thermal shift;
(b) the fourth day of mucus drying up or disappearance;
(c) the fourth day of the cervix closing or lowering.

2. *Rule C:* When all the signs do not coincide, the more conservative and safest course is to wait until all three of the above signs have been reached. However, almost the same results can be achieved by using either of the following two rules of thumb:

3. *Rule A* (more emphasis on temperatures): Phase III begins on the evening of the third day of full thermal shift crosschecked by at least two days of drying up or disappearance of the mucus.

4. *Rule B* (more emphasis on mucus): Phase III begins on the evening of the fourth day of drying up or dryness provided that is crosschecked by the temperature sign as follows:

(a) There are at least three days of temperatures above the pre-ovulation base.

(b) These temperatures are in a rising or elevated pattern.

(c) At least one of these temperatures has reached the normal thermal shift level of 4/10 of a degree above the pre-ovulation base.

The difference between the two rules above is that with Rule A *all* of the three temperatures constituting the thermal shift must be 4/10 of a degree above the pre-ovulation base. In Rule B, there must be three temperatures above the pre-ovulation base in a rising pattern but only one of these must be at the customary elevation of 4/10 of a degree. In both, the mucus symptom must have disappeared (or changed its consistency to the tacky type and largely disappeared in the cases of women who have mucus all the time).

Rule B assumes that the woman is well experienced in mucus observation. Because the mucus sign may be open to misinterpretation, inexperienced couples and those having the most serious reasons to avoid pregnancy should wait until all the signs coincide, or follow Rule A, or add at least one day to the figures in Rule B.

For Couples Using a Mucus-Only System

1. See Chapter 4.

2. Remember that mucus signs that are not corroborated by the thermal shift do not positively indicate postovulation infertility. Without such corroboration, it should be considered that more mucus and ovulation may occur later in the cycle.

Be aware of breakthrough bleeding and avoid any genital contact during any spotting, bleeding or menstruation.

Achieving a Pregnancy

If pregnancy is desired, ignore the preceding guidelines and have coitus on the days around the peak of mucus.

After Childbirth

• For the *Nursing* Mother—

1. If the natural infertility associated with breast-feeding is desired, follow the total mothering program outlined in Chapter 7.

2. Regard yourself as fertile after the return of menstruation, spotting, the appearance of clear, fertile-type mucus, and/or the feeling of vaginal wetness caused by such mucus.

3. Watch for the return of the mucus and cervix signs before the return of menstruation.

• For the *Non-nursing* Mother—

1. Refrain from coitus or genital contact until there are positive signs of the beginning of the postovulation infertility.

2. and 3. as above.

Special Guidelines for Couples
Just Learning the Sympto-thermal Method

• For Couples Serious About Avoiding Pregnancy—

1. Refrain from coitus for one cycle or at least until there is a clear sympto-thermal Rule A indication that Phase III has begun. One purpose of this advice is to assure that the woman can become acquainted with mucus observation without its being obscured by the residue of intercourse. Another is to avoid coitus during the relatively infertile phase, the time when inexperienced couples have the most surprise pregnancies.

2. Refrain from coitus and genital contact during the relatively infertile phase until enough experience is developed to apply the 21-day rule. This should be at least six months or more.

• For Couples Unwilling to Abide by the Previous Guideline and Willing to Accept a Slightly Greater Risk of Pregnancy—

1. Refrain from coitus in Phase I and II for at least two cycles so that the wife can gain a little experience in observing and interpreting the mucus and cervix signs of fertility and infertility.

2. Apply the 21-day rule cutoff as determined by whatever cycles you have records of. Or apply the guidelines for cycle days 4, 5 and 6 (Section A, Chapter 6). Thereafter, resume coital relations only after the sympto-thermal indication of the beginning of Phase III.

• For Couples Willing to Accept a Slightly Greater Risk Than Is Involved in the Above Guidelines —

1. Refrain from coitus in Phases I and II for at least one and preferably at least two cycles.

2. Use only the dry days for coitus.

3. On days past the end of Phase I as indicated by the 21-day rule, do not have coitus on consecutive days.

4. Once the mucus sign has appeared, refrain from coitus until the sympto-thermal indications of the beginning of Phase III.

Some Typical Examples

If you have understood the preceding pages, then it is very simple to review what your natural family planning will look like in a typical month. Let's go through several examples of different situations.

Couple A (a relaxed, combined system with coitus beyond the limits of the 21-day rule)

You are a couple who have two children, ages four and two. You are seriously considering having more children but would prefer to wait another year for the beginning of pregnancy. Mrs. A's shortest cycle has been twenty-seven days.

As Mrs. A, you will begin making and recording mucus observations as soon as your period has ended. You also begin taking and recording your temperature. You have noted that the 21-day rule would set day 6 as the last safe day. Trusting to your observations of mucus, you go beyond day 6 but do not have coitus on consecutive days.

As soon as you notice the mucus, you call your husband's attention to it. You both decide whether to accept pregnancy now or to limit your display of love and affection to non-genital ways. You discuss the matter long before going to bed. If you choose to avoid pregnancy, you avoid genital contact beginning with the first day of the show of cervical mucus. You notice that the mucus peaks in a few days in clearness and stretchability. You perhaps notice a little ovulation pain about this same time. Then, your temperature records start to show that your basal temperature is going up. You experience several "dry" days that coincide with a sustained higher temperature level. When the sympto-thermal signs indicate the beginning of Phase III, you resume coital relations with confidence that you can no longer become pregnant in this cycle. On the chart, you mark down the first day of your next period.

Aside from differences in family size, this will be the typical family planning process for many couples.

Couple B (using the 21-day rule)

You have serious reasons for wanting to avoid pregnancy at this time.

Therefore, you will play it safer than Couple A. For at least six months you have been limiting coitus to Phase III. During this six-month period you have kept temperature charts and have determined the length of your shortest cycle. Let us say you have a range from 26 to 30 days. Now you subtract 21 from the shortest cycle (26 in this case) and you have 5. Day 5 of your cycle is the last day on which you may have relations even if it and the next few days are "dry" days. Of course, if mucus is detectable on day 5 (which probably would indicate a shorter cycle), you would obviously not have genital contact on day 5.

What you have done is add a margin of safety. In a 26-day cycle, ovulation may occur as early as day 10 (26-16 = 10). If it occurred on day 10, mucus would probably be present on day 7, so you would avoid coitus then. By stopping on day 5, in this example, you will usually be stopping coital relations a day or several days before the beginning of mucus. (Remember that the cervical mucus both signals the approach of ovulation and helps sperm to live and unite with the ovum.) You will then wait until the mucus has peaked and dried and your temperature pattern has indicated three days of thermal shift. With the sympto-thermal indications of the beginning of Phase III, you may resume coital relations with the knowledge that the fertile stage has passed.

Couple C (very cautious)

You have what you consider the most serious reasons for avoiding pregnancy. Unless and until you are very experienced in observing, recording, and interpreting the mucus and cervix signs of ovulation, you will refrain from genital contact until *after* ovulation. That is, you will wait at least four days past the peak of your mucus and until the temperature record shows a thermal shift for at least three days. Once the thermal shift and mucus drying-up signs have been observed for that number of days, you are in the post-ovulatory phase. The chances of becoming pregnant in this phase are such that in one hundred years of childbearing age, you would have a surprise pregnancy in this phase less than once, an effectiveness about the same as the Pill.

Couple D (great irregularity)

No one is perfectly regular, having a built-in 28-day menstrual clock. Almost all women vary a normal one to four days each month. But when a woman varies from 20 days in one cycle to 45 days in the next cycle, she's irregular—and also an exceptional case. A few of these women may occasionally go for three months between menses. When a woman is highly irregular, it may be advisable to have a doctor check her endocrine functions.

Couple D, if they are serious about avoiding pregnancy, should refrain from genital contact until Phase III begins while Mrs. D learns how to observe the signs of mucus and cervix. If you are this couple, you will not have coitus during the menstrual flow for at least the first six months of charting. (In a very short cycle, ovulation might occur at or near the end of the menstrual flow.) In the next few cycles, while Mrs. D is becoming more experienced in detecting and recording the mucus and cervix signs of ovulation, you will refrain from genital contact until Phase III begins (as indicated by mucus, cervix, and the thermal shift sustained into the third day). Once Mrs. D has become experienced in detecting the mucus and cervix signs of ovulation, you will still refrain from the genital contact during the menstrual flow but can resume coital relations on the "mucus dry" and closed-cervix days after menstrual flow. However, you will not have coitus on consecutive days during Phase I. At the first sign of mucus or the opening or rising of the cervix, Couple D will recognize Phase II and will refrain from genital contact until the beginning of Phase III.

It should be apparent that one of the biggest advantages of the mucus and cervix signs is that they indicate the approach of ovulation. In a long cycle, sexual continence is normally not required for an extended period using these signs, while the couple who rely solely on the thermal shift that comes *after* ovulation may have a rather long period without coital relations.

Although it has been emphasized in previous chapters, we probably should repeat again that coitus prior to ovulation carries with it an inherently higher possibility of conception than coitus in the absolutely infertile stage for two reasons: (1) the possibility of not detecting the mucus or cervix signs, and (2) the possibility of extended sperm survival. For the experienced couple, the first possibility may be extremely small, but some couples with severe irregularity may find the guidelines for Couple C appropriate for them.

Couple E (menopause)

Mrs. E is approaching menopause. Her periods are becoming very irregular. She should use the mucus observations and the cervix signs as well as the basal temperatures. Then Couple E will follow the same type of pattern as Couple D.

Couple F (nursing mother)

This couple are new parents, and Mrs. F is nursing her baby according to the natural plan described briefly in this manual. Thus, her menstrual periods may not return for 6, 12, 20, or even 30 months.

Many couples who want only natural spacing between babies will ignore all signs of fertility and look forward to the next pregnancy. Others will decide to use the signs and temperature observation techniques only after the first menstruation.

In most cases, menstruation will occur before the first postpartum ovulation. However, many couples may not want to take the risk of being in that approximately 6 percent of cases in which the woman becomes pregnant before the first period. To reduce that risk, Mrs. F will begin looking for the pre-ovulation signs of mucus and the opening and/or rising of the cervix, especially after the baby has reached six months of age and is staying on solids. She may also begin temperature recordings. When she detects mucus, they will refrain from genital contact. If this is the true pre-ovulatory mucus, she will soon register a sustained rise on the temperature chart (see Chapter 7 for actual cases).

It should be noted that a mother's experience with one baby and postpartum menstruation is no guarantee of the same experience with the next baby and postpartum menustruation. For example, with baby 1 the mother may not ovulate until *after* her first postpartum menstruation, but with baby 2 she could ovulate *before* the first menstruation.

Concluding remarks

Several things are necessary for successful natural family planning, including motivation, proper instruction, adequate understanding, and cooperative attitudes. Through this manual and through its regular classes, the Couple to Couple League tries to assure proper instruction and adequate understanding. In several chapters and sprinkled throughout other sections are some ideas that can be used by a couple for their own motivation and attitude formation, but it is obvious that couples have to agree with these ideas and make them their own before they can be really helpful.

Undoubtedly, many couples experience occasional difficulties in the practice of natural family planning. However, with the proper attitudes, any such difficulties remain small ones and are turned into stepping stones toward increased marital maturity, mutual self-respect, and true sexual freedom.

In summary, the practice of natural family planning provides an extremely effective way of birth regulation. It does this not only without any harmful physical or psychological side effects but also provides its own benefits of developing the whole person and fostering marital maturity. With almost everybody recognizing the need for some form of birth regulation, and with almost everybody who commented upon

Watergate recognizing the need for character development and acting on principle, what's the world waiting for?

The authors hope this manual will serve your needs and prove helpful at every level.

APPENDIX I

Some reminders for beginners

A. Review

Cervix. (Review pages 45-48)
1. Examine the cervix daily at about the same time and in the same position.
2. During the infertile phases, especially in Phase III, the cervix is easier to reach and firm. As ovulation approaches, the cervix becomes harder to reach and becomes softer; the end of it opens a little, about the width of a finger tip.
3. Record cervix changes by using the symbols given on the chart such as the smaller and larger circles. (See page 68.)

Mucus. (Review pages 40-44, 48, 55-59, 74-77 and Appendix II.)
1. Check for mucus throughout the cycle and periodically during the day. Mark significant observations at the end of the day. Use symbols at bottom of chart. (See page 67.)
2. The most fertile type of mucus is described by different women in various ways: clear, cloudy, slippery, stretchy, like raw egg white, producing a feeling of vaginal wetness or lubrication.
3. If no mucus is noted, mark D for dry.

Temperature. (Review pages 49-54.)
1. Use a basal thermometer and take temperatures orally, rectally, or vaginally.
2. Take temperature for five minutes upon awakening, and take it at the same time each day. In case of a variation of $1/2$ hour or more, indicate the time on the chart. Read the thermometer and mark the reading on the chart. If temperature is between 2 lines on the thermometer, consistently use the lower reading. (See pages 66, 68, 69.)

Disturbances.
Disturbances in your normal routine such as a significant lack of sleep, alcohol the night before, or a cold may disturb your temperature, so note them on your chart. (See page 65.)

For all beginners. Refrain from coitus during Phase I and II. Even those trying to achieve pregnancy are advised to follow this guideline for a couple of cycles until the woman has gained some experience in mucus and cervix observations so she will know what to look for when fertility is returning after childbirth.

Counseling. Feel free to call your Teaching Couple. Those couples who are learning through self instruction may send charts to the national office at the address given in the front of this manual. Telephone counseling may be achieved by calling that office: (513) 661-7612.

B. Determining the beginning of Phase III, the time of post-ovulation infertility. (See pages 77-79)

Summary:
1. When all signs coincide, Phase III begins on the evening of the day indicated by
  a) the third day of full thermal shift;
  b) the fourth day of drying up or disappearance of mucus;
  c) the fourth day of the cervix closing and lowering.
New learners are advised to add one day to all of the above for at least the first two cycles to guard against possible misinterpretations.

2. When all the signs do *not* coincide, learners are advised to follow the more conservative course and to wait until at least the mucus and temperature guidelines have *both* been fulfilled. This means that there might be 4 or 5 (or more) days of apparent thermal shift before the 4th dry day is reached; or there might be 5 or 6 (or more) dry days before the 3rd day of thermal shift is reached. More experienced couples can follow the guidelines on page 78.

Coming off the pill. (See page 79 and figure 6.21.) The mucus sign may be of no help the first couple of cycles. It is recommended that a 5 day thermal shift be required to indicate the start of Phase III; this is to safeguard against possible misinterpretation of a temperature-only chart by an inexperienced couple.

Charting. (See Chapter 5.)

1. Draw lines as indicated in figures 5.2 and 6.1 to indicate your judgment about

    a) the pre-ovulation base

    b) the thermal shift level

    c) the end of Phase I and the beginning of Phase III.

2. Number at least 1) the first three days of thermal shift; 2) the first four days of drying up of the mucus, 3) the first four days of the closing of the cervix.

3. Keep a complete coitus record for yourselves. On charts that you hand in to CCL Teaching Couples, indicate at least the following coital record if you do not consider it an invasion of privacy:

    a) the last 2, if any, in Phase I

    b) any and all in Phase II. Please note if trying to achieve pregnancy, or taking chances, having a temporary change in plans, etc.

    c) first coitus in Phase III.

4. Note on your chart if coming off the pill, if breastfeeding or if there has been a recent childbirth or miscarriage.

C. Some reminders about Phase I for beginners:

1. Continence in Phase I is recommended during the first six cycles for three reasons:

    1) six cycles are required to apply the 21 day rule with reliability;

    2) Usually about 6 cycles are required for a woman to become well experienced in mucus and cervix signs;

    3) Continence in Phase I allows mucus observations to be made without the confusion frequently caused by seminal residue.

Couples unwilling to accept such continence should refer to page 198 for more relaxed guidelines, and review Section A of Chapter 6 for guidelines for cycle days 4, 5 and 6.

2. Experienced couples desiring to avoid pregnancy:

    1) Review the 21 day rule, pages 73-74.

    2) Review Detection of Mucus, pages 74-77.

    3) Review guidelines about menstruation and breakthrough bleeding, figure 6.7. Review summary of Phase I in Chapter 10.

D. A reminder for couples seeking to achieve pregnancy:

Review text for figure 6.2.

APPENDIX II
Developing Mucus Awareness
By Sheila Kippley

From talking with many women about the mucus observation, I think that many women check the mucus sign inadequately — only once a day or just before "possible" coitus or merely by what is seen. I have come to think that most women have not thoroughly learned the mucus observation until they become "aware" of its presence chiefly by external sensation. Seeing mucus on toilet paper is an additional aid but it is frequently not necessary in the overall picture of "becoming aware".

By becoming aware, I mean a woman learns that mucus is present as she wipes herself; without looking she feels upon wiping that the external surfaces of the vagina are wet and slippery. Or she suddenly feels wet while shopping, gardening or doing other ordinary day-to-day activities. We can compare our "becoming aware" to other observations. One who brushes her teeth after eating or has an apple or carrot develops a feeling for clean teeth. It bothers her to have sweets without any follow-up dental care as she has learned to dislike the feeling of "dirty" teeth. Again, a person easily becomes aware of the feeling of dry, clean skin as opposed to sweaty, sticky skin. A person who cooks "feels" the difference between water and oil and doesn't have to see them to note a difference.

When I was first learning mucus awareness, I felt I didn't have any mucus externally and that an internal exam was necessary to find anything at all. I didn't feel I could learn to rely upon the sensation of vaginal wetness or lubrication. I found later, however, that to learn this sensation it must be *thought about constantly* throughout the day *at first*. The best and easiest way to do this is for the woman to try to sense what she can feel when wiping herself because this is something every woman does now and then during the day. After a few months of this, she can make this observation almost automatically and without thinking. The observation is now well learned, and the woman has developed a simple body awareness of her fertility. As one who went from "no mucus" to 7 - 9 days of mucus prior to ovulation, I feel many other women *with effort at first* can also learn to sense their mucus on the days before ovulation.

There may be situations where the above may not prove practical. A woman with urinary leakage may feel wet almost all the time, but perhaps with experience, even many of these women can learn to distinguish an external slippery sensation during the mucus days. There may be other situations, especially among learners, where an internal exam may be much more informative, and certainly a woman should use the occasion of her cervix observation for mucus observation. However, the preceding comments have been intended to share what I and others have found to be helpful in making regular and accurate mucus observations.

* * *

The above article first appeared in the *CCL News* (Vol. I, No. 5; May-July, 1975). Various comments indicated that it proved very helpful to some women, so it is reproduced here. The *CCL News* provides helpful information in each issue and is sent free five times a year to all CCL members. Readers are thus urged to become members in order to keep well informed on new developments and insights. See introduction page xix for details.

Notes

208

Notes

Glossary of Terms

abortion. The destruction of a human life at any time between conception and birth. An abortion is called spontaneous when it occurs solely from natural causes; it is called induced when it results from human interference with the normal development of the unborn baby through the use of procedures, drugs, or devices designed to kill it.

abortifacient. A device or drug that causes an abortion.

absolutely infertile. Unable to become pregnant; refers to the infertility beginning several days after ovulation.

amenorrhea. Prolonged absence of menstrual periods.

anovulatory. Without ovulation; a menstrual cycle in which no ovulation occurs is anovulatory.

basal temperatures. The temperature of the human body at rest, unaffected by activity.

cervical mucus. A fluid secreted by glands in the cervix; it becomes watery and stretchy before and at the time of ovulation.

cervix. The lower, narrow part of the uterus.

coitus: Sexual intercourse.

coitus interruptus. Withdrawal from intercourse resulting in ejaculation outside the vagina.

coitus reservatus. Sexual intercourse controlled so that neither party experiences orgasm.

conception. The term applied to the creation of a new human life through the union of sperm and ovum; the process of becoming pregnant; fertilization.

condom. A contraceptive device put over the penis to prevent sperm from entering the vagina.

contraception. The practice of using procedures, devices, or drugs intended to prevent conception by interfering with the natural development or survival of ova and/or sperm either before or after ejaculation; artificial birth control.

contraceptives. Devices and drugs used in the practice of contraception.

corpus luteum. The name given to an ovarian follicle after it has released its ovum; as a gland, it secretes progesterone for about ten to fourteen days after ovulation.

diaphragm. A contraceptive device inserted into the vagina to cover the cervix to prevent sperm from entering it; called a cervical cap in England.

douche. A stream of water directed into the vagina to wash it out.

ecological breast-feeding. The type of nursing that fosters the natural relationship of mother and baby; characterized by (1) nursing as often as the baby wants; (2) no supplements or solids before the baby takes them from the family table; and (3) baby-led weaning.

ejaculation. The spasmodic expulsion of semen from the penis.

endocrine glands. Glands that secrete substances into the bloodstream for the purpose of controlling metabolism and other bodily functions.

endometrium. The inner lining of the uterus that builds up in each cycle and then is discharged in menstruation if no pregnancy occurred.

episiotomy. An incision made to enlarge the vaginal opening for birth.

estrogen. A hormone that causes the cervix to secrete mucus.

Fallopian tubes. The pair of tubes that conduct the egg from either ovary to the uterus.

fertile, fertility. In human reproduction, the state of the woman being able to conceive or of the man's sperm to fertilize the ovum.

follicle. Any one of thousands of tiny ovarian containers which each hold one ovum; upon release of its ovum, it becomes a gland called the corpus luteum.

FSH. Abbreviation for follicle stimulating hormone, a substance secreted by the pituitary gland to stimulate the maturation of ovarian follicles.

full thermal shift. Three or more temperatures *consecutively* at a level .4 (4/10) of 1° F. above the pre-ovulation base.

gynecologist. A medical doctor who specializes in the treatment of the female reproductive organs.

hormone. A glandular secretion that influences the action of cells in another part of the body.

implantation. The process of a newly conceived life at the blastocyst stage of development embedding in the lining of the uterus.

impotence. The inability to sustain an erection for coitus.

infertility. The state of a woman being unable to conceive or of a man to fertilize an ovum.

IUD. Abbreviation for intrauterine device, a device placed within the uterus to destroy human life prior to implantation.

labia. The lips, both inner and outer, of the vulva; the outermost parts of the female sexual organs.

lactation. The process of producing and yielding milk from the mammary glands.

luteal phase. The postovulation phase of the menstrual cycle under the influence of progesterone secreted from the corpus luteum.

luteinizing hormone (LH). A hormone secreted by the pituitary gland causing ovulation.

mammary glands. The breasts; more exactly, the glands in the breasts that secrete milk.

masturbation. Self-stimulation for carnal pleasure and orgasm.

menopause. The cessation of menstruation and ovarian activity.

menses. Synonym for menstruation.

menstruation. A vaginal bloody discharge caused by the sloughing off of the outer layers of the endometrium.

Minipill: A low-dosage oral contraceptive; a less powerful version of the Pill.

miscarriage. A spontaneous or natural abortion.

mittelschmerz. A German term meaning "pain in the middle" and used to describe a pain sometimes associated with ovulation.

mucorrhea. The state of producing cervical mucus.

mucus. A watery, slippery substance secreted by various mucus glands.

NFP. Abbreviation for natural family planning.

nocturnal emission. An involuntary and unconscious nighttime ejaculation of excess semen.

obstetrician. A medical doctor who specializes in the delivery of babies and in pre- and postnatal care of the mother.

os. The Latin word for mouth; the opening of the cervix.

ovary. The female reproductive organ containing the ova, or eggs.

ovulation. The process of an ovarian follicle releasing its ovum, thus making the woman fertile and able to become pregnant.

ovum (plural: ova). The woman's egg.

pediatrician. A medical doctor who specializes in the treatment of children.

penis. The male sexual organ used for coitus.

Pill. Capitalized, it refers to all the various oral contraceptive pills.

pituitary gland. A gland located at the base of the brain that controls many bodily functions through various secretions.

postpartum. After childbirth.

premenopause. The stage in life between the years of normal fertility and menopause.

pre-ovulation base. The level from which the thermal shift is measured; usually determined by the normal highs among the pre-shift six temperatures.

pre-shift six. The six temperatures immediately before the beginning of the rising temperatures that make up the thermal shift.

progesterone. A female hormone secreted by the corpus luteum.

prostate gland. A male sexual organ that provides a fluid which mixes with sperm to produce semen.

rhythm method. A term used to describe calendar rhythm, a system of estimating fertility based on previous cycle lengths.

rules of thumb. See Chapter 6, Section A for a description of the basic rules of thumb.

scrotum. The sac below the penis that contains the testicles.

sperm. The male cells that unite with the female ovum to cause conception.

sterilization. The process of rendering either male or female sterile, i.e., incapable of becoming pregnant or causing pregnancy.

sympto-thermal method. A natural family planning system making use of all the signs of fertility.

testicles. The male sexual organs contained in the scrotum and producing sperm.

thermal shift. The postovulation rise in temperatures sustained in an overall rising or elevated pattern for at least three days, reaching and staying at a level usually .4 (4/10) of 1° F. above the pre-ovulation base. See also "full thermal shift."

tubal ligation. A sterilization procedure consisting of tying the Fallopian tubes to prevent sperm from meeting ova.

tubal pregnancy. Ectopic pregnancy; a pregnancy in which implantation occurs within the Fallopian tube rather than in the uterus.

uterus. The female organ in which the baby grows during the nine months of pregnancy; frequently called the womb.

vagina. The female sexual organ used in coitus.

vaginal foams and jellies. Chemical contraceptive products made to be inserted in the vagina before coitus to kill sperm.

vasectomy. A male sterilization procedure that prevents sperm from becoming part of the semen.

vulva. The external parts of the female sexual organs, including the labia.

womb. The uterus.

Bibliography

A special note of thanks is due to Jeffrey J. Pitman, who in 1972 presented the authors with a 92-item annotated bibliography he had developed to fulfill a library science project requirement. (The project was to prepare a bibliography on a subject about which it was difficult to find information. Mr. Pitman chose natural family planning.) Without that base, the current bibliography simply would not exist in its present form. To Mr. Pitman's project we have added other items and deleted a few. Because in the final list we have not distinguished his contributions from our own, we assume responsibility for all of the annotations.

The bibliography is not complete. We have limited ourselves to scientific treatments of the ovulation mechanism that are directly related to natural family planning. Further references to scientific articles will be found in the bibliographies appended to the works listed herein. Several of these articles have been listed without annotation. The overall subject of birth control philosophy is so vast that it would take an entire book to begin a bibliography. The material presenting a case for the natural-methods-only approach to conception regulation, however, is much more limited. Those wanting to pursue or research the philosophy behind natural family planning will find the present list fairly complete. Several entries represent a diametrically opposed philosophy and are included because they are referred to in the text of this book.

Albury, W. R., and Richard J. Connell. "Humanae Vitae and the Ecological Argument." *Laval theblogique et philosophique*, XXVII (June, 1971), pp. 135-149.
    An attack by Mr. Albury on Mr. Connell's "A Defense of Humanae Vitae" (see Connell entry) and a reply by Mr. Connell, who also formalizes the main arguments in the article under attack.

Bartzen, Peter J. "Effectiveness of the Temperature Rhythm System of Contraception." *Child and Family* (Spring, 1969), pp. 108-118.
    Data received from 441 women. Characteristics of the patients, difficulties of the system, and results achieved. The types of and reasons for failures. Reprinted from *Fertility and Sterility,* 18 (1967), pp. 694-706.

Beebe, G. W. *Conception and Fertility in the Southern Appalachians.* Baltimore: Williams and Wilkins, 1942.
    Reports finding a pregnancy rate of 3 per 100 women-years of exposure during lactation amenorrhea. Not personally reviewed.

Bergman, P. "Sexual Cycle, Time of Ovulation and Time of Optimal Fertility in Woman." *Acta. Obstet. Gynaec. Scand.,* 29 (1950), Supp. IV.

214

Billings, E. L. and John J., J. B. Brown, and H. G. Burger. "Symptoms and Hormonal Changes Accompanying Ovulation." *Lancet* (February 5, 1972), pp. 282-284.

Reports results of a study on hormonal changes accompanying ovulation; relates them to observation of changes in cervical mucus.

Billings, John J. *Natural Family Planning: The Ovulation Method.* Collegeville: The Liturgical Press, 1973 (2nd American edition), 38 pp.

In this edition, Dr. Billings advocates the mucus symptom alone as sufficient for fertility awareness and criticizes the use of the basal temperatures as unnecessary.

———— *The Ovulation Method.* Los Angeles: Borromeo Guild, 1972 (1st American edition), 99 pp.

Describes the mucus-only approach to fertility awareness with some correlation with basal temperatures.

———— and Evelyn L., and Maurice Caterinich. *Atlas of the Ovulation Method.* Melbourne, Australia: Advocate Press, 1973. 33 pp.

Intended as a teacher's companion to *The Ovulation Method,* 4th edition (Australia).

———— and Evelyn L. "Determination of Fertile and Infertile Days by the Mucus Pattern: Development of the Ovulation Method." *Proceedings of a Research Conference on Natural Family Planning.* Washington: The Human Life Foundation, 1973, pp. 149-163, plus discussion, pp. 164-170.

Describes rationale and key elements of the mucus-only system of fertility awareness.

Blackall, Randall. *Design for Marriage.* Hamden, Conn.: Cana House, 1966. 105 pp.

Periodic abstinence is considered within the context of the entire marriage. Discusses the various forms that communication between husband and wife can take, and how to use each to its best advantage.

Boutselis, J., N. Vorys and J. Ullery. "Regulation of Ovulation Time in Normal Women with Clomiphene Citrate and Perfecting the Practice of the Rhythm Method." *Linacre,* XXXII (November, 1966), pp. 349-352.

Brayer, Franklin T., Leonard Chiazze, Jr. and Benedict J. Duffy. "Calendar Rhythm and Menstrual Cycle Range." *Fertility and Sterility,* Vol. 20, No. 2 (1969), pp. 279-288.

Shows difficulties of using calendar rhythm because of cycle range.

Brown, J. B., S. C. MacLeod, C. MacNaughton, M. A. Smith and B. Smyth. "A Rapid Method for Measuring Oestrogens in Human Urine Using a Semi-automatic Extractor," *Journal of Endocrinology,* Vol. 42 (1968), p. 5.

Cantrelle, P., and H. Leridon. "Breast-feeding, Mortality in Childhood and Fertility in a Rural Zone of Senegal." *Population Studies,* Vol. 25, No. 3 (1971), pp. 505-533.

A study of women who nursed for 12 months, for 24 months, and for 36 months. When weaning occurs between 12 and 36 months, there is an additional 9 months of spacing for every 1 year of nursing.

Capon, Robert Farrar. *Bed and Board: Plain Talk About Marriage.* New York: Simon and Schuster, 1965. 172 pp.

An Episcopal priest talks openly about marriage. Explains religious difficulty of accepting contraception.

Connell, Richard J. "A Defense of Humanae Vitae." *Laval theblogique et philosophique,* Vol. XXVI (February, 1970), pp. 57-87.
Considers the nature of man, moral issues in contraception, and the regulation of births.

Costanzo, Joseph F. "Academic Dissent: An Original Ecclesiology." *The Thomist,* Vol. XXXIV, No. 4 (October, 1970), pp. 636-653.
A critical review of two books by theologians dissenting from Humanae Vitae.

————— "Papal Magisterium, Natural Law and Humanae Vitae." *American Journal of Jurisprudence,* Vol. 16 (1971), pp. 259-289.
A defense of the doctrine of marital non-contraception in terms of natural law and church history.

Cox, R. T. "Gas-chromotography in the Analysis of Urinary Pregnanediol." *Journal of Chromatography,* Vol. 12 (1963), p. 242.

Cronin, T. J. "Influence of Lactation Upon Ovulation." *Lancet,* Vol. II (August 24, 1968), pp. 422-424.

Dalsace, Jean, and Raoul Palmer. *La Contraception.* Paris: Presses Universitaires de France, 1966. 204 pp.
An introduction to the advantages and disadvantages of various methods of regulating conception from a biological and psychological viewpoint. Not personally examined.

Daly, Bernard, and Mae Daly. "Knowledge: Key to Conjugal Love." *Marriage* (October, 1970), pp. 52-57.
Why a couple should have knowledge of the basic pattern of the fertility-infertility cycle and its role in their marriage.

D'Arcy Hart, Ruth. "Monthly Rhythms of Libido in Married Women." *British Medical Journal,* Vol. I (April 2, 1960), pp. 1023-1024.
A majority of married women experience an increase in libido around menstruation. A large minority have no monthly rhythm of libido. Less than 5 percent have an increase in sexual desire at ovulation.

Davis, E. Edward. "The Clinical Use of Oral Basal Temperatures." *Journal of the American Medical Association,* Vol. CXXX (April 6, 1946), pp. 929-932.
Basal temperatures, their relation to ovulation, and their use in avoiding conception.

Davis, Morris Edward. *Natural Child Spacing.* New York: Hanover House, 1953. 67 pp.
A description of the temperature method of family planning with illustration and diagrams.

Derrick, Christopher, *Honest Love and Human Life.* New York: Coward-McCann, Inc., 1969. 158 pp.
A supporter of Humanae Vitae explains why he thinks that contraception is dishonest. Derrick examines the population explosion and tells why he regards man's essential choice as one between widespread discipline and control and widespread disaster.

Dewan, E. M. "On the Possibility of a Perfect Rhythm Method of Birth Control by Periodic Light Stimulation." *American Journal of Obstetrics and Gynecology,* Vol. 99 (1967), p. 1016.

————"Rhythms." *Science and Technology* (January 1969), p. 20.

Doring, Gerhard K. "Detection of Ovulation by the Basal Body Temperature Method." *Proceedings of a Research Conference on Natural Family Planning;* Washington: The Human Life Foundation, 1973, pp. 171-189.

Explains that "the use of the Temperature Method is based on the experience that there has never been a conception from the third day of the hyperthermic phase of the cycle until the following menstruation" (p. 172).

————*Die Termperaturemethode zur Emphangnisverhutung.* Thieme, Stuttgart, 1 Ed. 1954; 7 Ed. 1968.

———— "Temperaturmessung als einfaches Hilfsmittel zur Zyklusanalyse." *Geburtsch. Frauenheilk,* Vol. 9 (1949), p. 757.

———— "Uber die Bestimmung des Ovulationstermines mit Hilfe der rhythmischen Schwankungen von Atmung und Korpertemperatur." *Klin. Wschr.,* Vol. 27 (1949), p. 309.

———— "Uber die Zuverlassigkeit der Temperaturmethode zur Empfangnisverhutung." *Deutsche Medizinische Wochenschrift.* 92:23 (June, 1967), pp. 1055-1061. Abstracted in English in the 1968 *Yearbook of Obstetrics and Gynecology,* J. B. Greenhills, ed. Chicago: Yearbook Medical Publishers, Inc., 1968, p. 354.

Reports a very high level of effectiveness among 996 women who used the basal temperature system from 4 to 19 years (96-99 percent levels of effectiveness depending on how the system was used).

Doyle, Joseph. "Culdotomy for Observation of Tube Ovarian Physiology at Ovulation Time." *Fertility and Sterility,* II (November-December, 1951), pp. 475-486.

Observation of the rupture of the follicle and the formation of the corpus luteum in correlation with basal body temperature, showing basal body temperature to be correct in determining ovulation.

———— et al. "The New Fertility Testing Tape." *Journal of the American Medical Association,* Vol. CLXXII (April 16, 1960), pp. 1744-1750.

An explanation of the test for glucose in mucus from the cervix to determine ovulation. How the testing tape works and details of the technique.

Dunn, H. P. "The Safe Period." *Lancet,* Vol. II (September 1, 1956), pp. 441-442.

A report on the use of calendar rhythm by 156 women. the results they achieved and the failure rates given according to type: total failure rate, patient failure rate, and method failure rate.

———— "The Reliability of the Safe Period." *Child and Family* (Fall, 1968), pp. 305-310.

Scientific reports on the reliability of the safe period are compared to each other and to the reliability of other methods of conception control. The reasons for the large variations of reliability reported for the rhythm method are explained.

Eastman, Nicholas J. Editorial comments. *Obstetrical and Gynecological Survey,* 10:5 (1955), pp. 661-662.

Notes the child-spacing effect of ecological breast-feeding. Where breast-feeding infertility is the sole means of conception postponement, an average of less than eight children will be born to women who marry between the ages of 20 and 24.

Eastman, Nicholson. "The Effect of the Interval Between Births on Maternal and Fetal Outlook." *Child and Family* (Fall 1969), pp. 323-348.
A study of what is the best interval between pregnancies for both mother and child. The effect of artificial spacing on this interval.

Elstein, Max. "The Detection of Ovulation." *Proceedings of the Royal Society of Medicine,* Vol. LVIII (November, 1965), p. 910.
The correlation between basal body temperature, vaginal smear, and endometrical biopsy in determining ovulation.

Ewers, Frank. "Scientific Rhythm." *Linacre,* Vol. XXXII (August, 1965), pp. 251-257.
An explanation of four methods of finding ovulation: basal body temperature, oral saliva test, cervical glucose test, and spinnbarkeit test. A comparison of their effectiveness.

Firestone, Shulamith. *The Dialectic of Sex: The Case for Feminist Revolution.* New York: William Morrow, 1970. 274 pp.
Inter alia, argues for the doing away with marriage now that efficient contraception is at hand.

Foster, Raymond et al. "Salivary Alkaline Phosphatase Levels During the Menstrual Cycle." Paper presented at the American Chemical Society National Meeting, Washington, D.C., September 17, 1971.
Examines the relationship between alkaline phosphatase activity and ovulation. Establishes the feasibility of a test system utilizing the alkaline phosphatase levels in saliva to predict ovulation.

Francoeur, Robert T. *Eve's New Rib: Twenty Faces of Sex, Marriage and Family.* New York: Harcourt, Brace, Jovanovich, 1972. 253 pp.
Presents 20 types of sexual living arrangements made possible by efficient contraception; only one is monogamous marriage.

Frankl, Victor. *Man's Search for Meaning.* New York: Washington Square Press, Inc., 1963. 214 pp.
In this "Introduction to Logotherapy," Frankl shows how suffering can help in the discovery of meaning in life.

Fried, John J. "The Incision Decision." *Esquire* (June, 1972), p. 118 ff.
Describes factors to be considered before having a vasectomy.

Geller, Sacha. *The Temperature Guide for Women.* London: The Pitman Press, 1969. 81 pp.
Discusses the ovarian cycle—its phases and relationship to the menstrual cycle; how to distinguish the ovarian cycle from the temperature curve; and practical mechanics of the temperature method and some difficulties that may be foreseen.

Georg, I.E. *The Truth About Rhythm.* New York: P. J. Kennedy and Sons, 1962. 212 pp.
Explanation of the female cycle, its variations and patterns, and the practical application of the temperature method to avoid conception.

Greenblatt, Robert B. *Ovulation*. Philadelphia: J. P. Lippincott Company, 1966. 341 pp.
   A medical work on the physiology and pathology of ovulation and its relationship to pregnancy. Chapter 26 is specifically concerned with detecting ovulation to avoid pregnancy.

Guttmacher, Alan F. "Fertility of Man." *Fertility and Sterility*, 3:4 (1952), pp. 281-289.
   Reports on findings about birth rates among populations practicing no form of conception regulation and among breast-feeding mothers.

Gioiosa, Rose. "Incidence of Pregnancy During Lactation in 500 Cases." *American Journal of Obstetrics and Gynecology,* Vol. LXX (July-December, 1955), pp. 162-174.
   The degree of protection against pregnancy offered by lactation analyzed for each month after birth.

————— "Breast-feeding and Child Spacing." *Child and Family* (Spring, 1964), pp. 1-8.
   A comparison of the results and conclusions of various research studies regarding breast-feeding and child spacing.

Guy, Francois and Michele. *Comment aider un foyer a comprender la courbe thermique*. Ile Maurice, France: Rose Hille, 1966. 148 pp.
   How to help married couples understand the temperature curve correctly, written by a husband-and-wife doctor team. Includes a guide to many samples of the temperature curve. Not personally examined.

Hartman, Carl G. *Science and the Safe Period*. London: Balliere, Tindall and Cos, Ltd., 1962. 294 pp.
   An explanation of the physiology behind the Ogino-Knaus method of calculating the fertile and infertile days in women.

Hilgers, Thomas W. "The Intrauterine Device: Contraceptive or Abortifacient?" *Marriage and Family Newsletter,* Vol. 5, Nos. 1, 2, 3 (January-March 1974), entire issue. And in *Minnesota Medicine* (June 1974), pp. 493-501.
   Reviews the medical literature and concludes that "the primary action of the IUD must be classed as abortifacient."

Hillabrand, John. "Rhythm: II. Natural Family Planning." *Child and Family* (Winter 1969), pp. 2-4.
   The advantages and efficacy of natural family planning are considered. The view is presented that the implications and consequences of each conception control method must be considered before it can be judged.

Hillebrand, Wilhelm. *Geburtsch Frauenheilk,* Vol. 20 (1960), p. 188. (See also *Journal of Biosocial Science,* Vol. 3 [1971], p. 331.)
   By the German Catholic priest who was the first to use the fluctuations of the female body temperature to determine the infertile days. Not personally reviewed.

Hollender, Marc H. "Women's Wish to Be Held: Sexual and Nonsexual Aspects." *Medical Aspects of Human Sexuality,* (October 1971), pp. 12-26.
   States that in some women the desire to be held and cuddled is the major sexual aim and not just foreplay.

Holt, Jan Gerard. *La Fertilite'Cyclique de la femme.* Paris: Vigot Frères, 1959. 80 pp.

Discusses the periodic fertility of women and a method of regulating conception based on the shortest cycle and temperature reading. Not personally examined.

Holt, J. G. H. *Marriage and Periodic Abstinence.* London: Longman's, 1961. 86 pp.

The theory of periodicity in fertility. The syndrome of ovulation. A comparison of techniques for determining ovulation by the chief of obstetrics and gynecology at the University of Utrecht.

Geburtenregulung auf biologischem Wege. Vienna: Deuticke, 1959.

Huxley, Aldous. *Brave New World.* New York: Harper and Row, 1969 (first published in 1932).

Huxley's novel showing a society built on contraception, no marriage, sex-with-anyone, no religion, and relief of tension through drugs.

Jacobi, Mary. *The Question of Rest for Women During Menstruation.* Boylston Prize, 1876. New York: G. P. Putnams, 1877.

An American woman provides the first exact description of changes in female body temperatures during the rhythm of the menstrual cycle.

Johnson, Arthur, and Connie Johnson. "Serena." *Marriage* (May, 1968), pp. 6-12.

A description of Serena, a Canadian-based natural family planning organization. How the temperature method works and some of its psychological aspects. What people think about rhythm and what it actually is.

Joyce, Mary. "The Sexual Revolution Is Yet to Begin." T. W. Hilgers and D. J. Horan, eds., *Abortion and Social Justice.* New York: Sheed and Ward, 1972, pp. 221-229.

The real sexual revolution will begin when genital intercourse is regarded as an option, not a necessity, for sexual freedom.

———— *Love Responds to Life.* Kenosha, Wisc.: Prow, 1971. 144 pp.

An explanation of Humanae Vitae that proceeds on a philosophical level. A discussion of the nature of love, the unity of the person, and sexual freedom.

———— *The Meaning of Contraception.* Staten Island, N.Y.: Alba House, 1970. 148 pp.

A reinterpretation and analysis of the natural law and its relationship to contraception. It examines coitus from both metaphysical and physical points of view, and looks at conception control from a view of the nature of the total human being.

———— and Robert Joyce. *New Dynamics in Sexual Love.* Collegeville, Minn.: St. John's University Press, 1970. 182 pp.

A married couple show how the meanings of human love and sexuality are truly inexhaustible. They discuss marriage of the future and present a philosophy of sexual love.

Kanaby, Donald, and Helen Kanaby. *Sex, Fertility and the Catholic.* Staten Island, N.Y.: Alba House, 1965. 144 pp.

A Catholic couple describe rhythm as they practiced it, discuss its biological and psychological aspects, and the problems that they faced.

220

Included are sixteen of their "irregular" charts and how they were interpreted.

Keefe, Edward. "A Practical Open-Scale Thermometer for Timing Human
Ovulation." *New York State Medical Journal,* Vol. II (November 1, 1949),
pp. 2554-2555.
The development of the Ovulindex thermometer, used in measurement of
temperatures to find the time of ovulation, and how it differs from a regular
thermometer.

Keefe, Edward F. "The Cervix, A Guide to Systematic Abstinence." *Coverline.*
(Spring, 1970), pp. 1-2.
New findings to update his 1962 article regarding physical changes in the
cervix. How to apply cervix signs to determine ovulation.

———— "Self-Observation of the Cervix to Distinguish Days of Possible Fertility." *Bulletin of the Sloane Hospital for Women,* Vol. VIII (December,
1962), pp. 129-136.
Sensory changes of size, texture, and mucus in the cervix that may be determined by the woman as an aid to fertility control.

Kimball, Robbins E. "How I Get Mothers to Breast-feed." *Physicians Management* (June, 1968).
Notes that breast-fed babies are comparatively healthier than bottle-fed
babies.

Kippley, John F. "Catholic Sexual Ethics: The Continuing Debate on Birth
Control." *Linacre,* 41:1 (February, 1974), pp. 8-25.
Uses reasons advanced by the dissenters to show that dissent from the
Catholic Hospital Directives and Humanae Vitae is no longer valid; shows
practical import for Catholic physicians.

———— "Continued Dissent: Is It Responsible Loyalty?" *Theological Studies,*
32:1 (March, 1971), pp. 48-65.
Shows that the theology of dissent has used premises that logically entail
dissent from the entirety of the traditional sexual ethic or any part of it.

———— *Covenant, Christ and Contraception.* Staten Island, N.Y.: Alba House,
1970. 160 pp.
A defense of the doctrine of marital non-contraception through a personalistic approach based on the couple's covenant in marriage. The difference between contraception and periodic abstinence is explained.

———— "Holy Communion: Eucharistic and Marital." *Ave Maria* (February 25,
1967), pp. 9-12.
Draws parallels between attitudes and dispositions for valid participation
in the Eucharist and in coitus.

———— and Sheila K. Kippley. "The Relation Between Breast-feeding and
Amenorrhea." *Journal of Obstetrical, Gynecological and Neo-Natal Nursing,*
1:4 (November-December, 1972), pp. 15-21.
Reports on a survey showing that a certain type of breast-feeding and baby
care (not the typical American forms) provide, on the average, over a year's
postpartum absence of menstrual periods.

Kippley, Sheila K. *Breast-feeding and Natural Child Spacing: The Ecology of
Natural Mothering.* New York: Harper and Row, 1974. Penguin, 1975.
197 pp.

Describes the type of mothering and baby care that normally produces an extended period of postpartum infertility. Contains extensive references to the literature on lactation amenorrhea.

Knaus, Hermann. *Periodic Fertility and Sterility in Woman.* Trans. by F. H. A. Marshall. Vienna: Wilhelm Maudrich, 1934. 162 pp.
The biological basis of periodic fertility and the calendar determination of fertile and sterile periods; a summation of all the papers on the subject presented by the co-discoverer of the idea.

———— "Uber den Zeitpunkt ker Konzeptionsfahigkeit des Weibes." *Munch. Med. Wschr.,* 76:1167 (1929).

Koep, Dennis M. "Christian Marriage." *Coverline* (March-April, 1967), pp. 1-3.
The problem of love and control in marriage. Periodic continence: what it takes, what it means, and some of its advantages.

La Leche League International. *The Womanly Art of Breast-feeding.* Franklin Park, Ill.: La Leche League International, 1963. 166 pp.
All aspects of breast-feeding are covered in this book, but Chapters 1 and 4 contain specific material on how breast-feeding affects menstruation and ovulation.

Lamm, Norman. "The New Morality and the Tradition of Periodic Abstinence in Jewish Law." *Child and Family* (Summer 1969), pp. 196-210.
The Jewish tradition of periodic abstinence. The new morality and the Jewish view of sexuality. The value of abstinence in Jewish tradition and its effect on family life.

Lanctot, Claude. "Effectiveness Studies of Temperature Rhythm Family Planning." *Coverline,* Section I (Summer, 1971), pp. 1-2; Section II (Fall, 1971), pp. 1-2,5.
Section I explains the various applications of the temperature method, how to calculate effectiveness, and the different types of failure rates. Section II provides a summary of the results of nine different studies and analyses the failure rates.

———— and Anne. "Reliability of the Sympto-thermic Method." *Coverline* (January-February, 1968), pp. 2-3.
Summaries and descriptions of recent studies.

———— and Suzanne Parenteau-Carreau. "Studies of the Effectiveness of Temperature Methods of Family Planning." *Proceedings of a Research Conference on Natural Family Planning.* Washington, D.C.: The Human Life Foundation, 1973, pp. 311-316.
Summarizes the findings of various effectiveness studies.

Lass, Paul M. "Studies Relating to Time of Human Ovulation." *Endocrinology,* Vol. XXIII (July, 1938), pp. 39-43.
A study of ovulation during lactation regarding anovulatory and ovulatory cycles.

Latz, Leo J., and Emil Reiner. "Further Studies on the Sterile and Fertile Periods in Women." *American Journal of Obstetrics and Gynecology,* Vol. XLIII (January, 1942), pp. 74-77.

Levin, Max. "Sexual Fulfillment in the Couple Practicing Rhythm." *Child and*

Family (Winter 1969), pp. 5-13.
The quality of the marriage itself is said to be the determining factor is sexual fulfillment. The character of the man and woman entering marriage and its relationship to sexual fulfillment is considered.

────── "Sexual Fullfillment with Rhythm." *Marriage* (June, 1966), pp. 32-35.
Periodic continence: an obstacle to marital love? Continence and its relation to a sound marriage.

Lippmann, Walter. *A Preface to Morals.* New York: Macmillan, 1929.
Inter alia, links contraception with other, more recognized sexual disorders.

Loh, H. C., and C. W. M. Wilson. "Relationship of Human Ascorbic-Acid Metabolism to Ovulation." *Lancet* (January 16, 1971), pp. 110-112.
A study showing that the ascorbic acid excretion of an ovulating woman reaches a peak three days prior to ovulation, and also increases at the time of ovulation. Results compared with basal body temperature.

Lynch, William. *Marriage Manual for Catholics.* New York: Trident Press, 1964. 359 pp.
The president of the staff of St. Mary's Hospital in Boston devotes Chapter 9 to limitation of the family, discussing the use of periodic continence and its problems, and how to chart the temperature curve.

McCann, Joan. "The Saliva Test." *Marriage* (September, 1969), pp. 4-7.
An explanation of the saliva test as a means to determine time of ovulation.

Marshall, John. "A Field Trial of the Basal Body Temperature Method of Regulating Births." *Lancet,* Vol. II (July 6, 1968), pp. 8-10.
A study of the biological effectiveness of the temperature method as used by 500 couples. Results are considered both overall and with the test group broken into several subcategories.

────── *The Infertile Period.* 2nd ed. Baltimore: Helicon Press, 1967. 120 pp.
The clinical neurologist of the University of London explains the physiological principles behind the infertile period. Instructions in the temperature method are provided, and special circumstances that may arise are given attention. The physiological aspects and effectiveness of the infertile period are discussed.

────── *Catholics, Marriage and Contraception.* Baltimore: Helicon Press, 1965, 212 pp.
A historical, theological, and medical analysis of contraception from the Catholic viewpoint. Chapters 6, 8, and 9 concern periodic continence in particular.

────── *Planning for a Family.* London: Faber and Faber, 1965. 159 pp.
By a series of charts the author shows the changes of temperature which occur during the menstrual cycle.

────── "Thermal Changes in the Normal Menstrual Cycle." *British Medical Journal,* Vol. I (January 12, 1963), pp. 102-110.
A study of the rise in basal body temperature due to ovulation. The duration of the postovulatory phase and its relation to total cycle length.

────── and B. Rowe. "Psychologic Aspects of the Basal Body Temperature Method of Regulating Births." *Fertility and Sterility,* Vol. XXI (January,

1970), pp. 14-19.

An analysis of statistics gathered from 410 couples using the temperature method of periodic continence regarding the psychological effects of that method.

Marshall, John R. "Prediction, Detection and Control of Ovulation: An Overview." *Proceedings of a Research Conference on Natural Family Planning.* Washington, D.C.: The Human Life Foundation, 1973, pp. 135-148.

A review of research on ovulation. Contains a 64-item bibliography on technical works, most of which are not included in the present bibliography.

Martin, Purvis. "Detection of Ovulation by the Basal Temperature Curve with Correlating Endometrial Studies." *American Journal of Obstetrics and Gynecology,* Vol. XXXXVI (July-December, 1943), pp. 53-62.

Marx, Paul. *The Death Peddlers: War on the Unborn.* Collegeville, Minn.: St. John's University Press, 1971. 191 pp.

Reports on what took place at the Symposium on Implementation of Therapeutic Abortion in Los Angeles, January 22-24, 1971. Provides insights into the plans of the advocates of abortion.

Mintz, Morton. *The Pill: An Alarming Report.* Boston: Beacon Press, 1970.

Reports on the side effects of the oral contraceptives.

Moore, W. M. "Ovulation Symptoms and Avoidance of Conception." *Lancet* (March 11, 1972), p. 588.

Notes there is no solid evidence for a second ovulation occurring some time after the first one.

Moore, W. M. O. "The Mauritius Experience." *Child and Family* (Spring, 1969, pp. 102-107.

The use of the temperature method of family planning on a national scale in Mauritius to check that country's population growth. How the program was operated and its results. Reprinted from *Fertility and Sterility,* 18 (1967), pp. 694-706.

Muller, Paul, and G. C. Nabors. "Making Rhythm Work." *Marriage* (June, 1964), pp. 8-18.

Divided into two parts. Section I discusses natural family planning from a general viewpoint of family limitation, giving basic biological information and discussing the problem of motivation. Section II describes the temperature method proper.

Murphy, John F., and John D. Laux. *The Rhythm Way to Family Happiness.* New York: Hawthorn Books, Inc., 1967. 200 pp.

An explanation of the calendar method of rhythm. Tables showing how to find the fertile period for any size variation between longest and shortest cycle at any time during the year.

Nabors, Grover C. "A Doctor's View of Rhythm." *Marriage* (September, 1968), pp. 42-44.

A gynecologist discusses the sexual desire of women, and whether or not that desire has any relation to distinct periods of the menstrual cycle. The effect of abstention on sexual desire.

———— "Speak Up: A Doctor's View of Rhythm." *Child and Family* (Winter, 1969), pp. 14-15.

Difficulty with rhythm—whether a cause or symptom of difficulties in the marriage. Sexual desire and abstention. Frustration and rhythm. Whether there are biological periods of greater or lesser sexual desire in women.

Nolen, William A. "Vasectomy: A Cautionary Note." *McCalls* (June 1972), p. 136.
Cautions against vasectomy as a means of relieving marital tension due to fear of pregnancy.

Noonan, John T., Jr. *Contraception: A History of Its Treatment by the Catholic Theologians and Canonists.* Cambridge, Mass.: Harvard University Press, 1965. 561 pp.
The classic on the subject indicated by the subtitle.

Ogino, Kyusaku. "Historical Studies on Corpora Lutea, Period of Ovulation, Relation Between Corpora Lutea and Cyclic Changes in Uterine Mucous Membrane, and the Period of Fertilization." *Japanese Medical World,* 8 (1928), p. 147.

Palmer, Allan. "The Diagnostic Use of the Basal Body Temperature in Gynecology and Obstetrics." *Obstetrical and Gynecological Survey,* Vol. IV (February, 1949), pp. 1-26.
The historical background of the basal body temperature. How to take the temperature, and interpretation of the temperature curves to understand the ovulatory and menstrual changes taking place.

Palmer, R. "Evaluation des méthodes de contraception basées sur l'abstinence périodique et en particulier la méthode des températures." In *La Contraception.* Paris: Masson, 1963.

Pascal, Juliette. "Some Aspects of Post-Partum Physiology: Contribution of the Basal Body Temperature and Its Application to Birth Regulation. A Statistical Study of 750 Cases." Unpublished M. D. dissertation, University of Nancy, 1969. 310 pp.

Pearl, R. "Contraception and Fertility in 2,000 Women." *Human Biology,* 4 (1932), p. 363.

Peel, John, and Malcolm Potts. *Textbook of Contraceptive Practice.* New York: Cambridge University Press, 1969.
Inter alia, describes "breakthrough ovulation" among women taking oral contraceptives (p. 99).

Prem, Konald A. "Temperature Method in the Practice of Rhythm." *Child and Family* (Fall, 1968), pp. 311-327.
A description of the temperature method with reasons for apparent failures explained. Article is not up to date with Dr. Prem's current method of instruction.

Racy, John. "Ten Misuses of Sex." *Medical Aspects of Human Sexuality* (February, 1971), pp. 136-145.
Explains ten motivations for intercourse that the psychiatrist-author finds less than normal.

Ratner, Herbert. "Child-Spacing: I. Man Against Nature." *Child and Family* (Fall, 1969), pp. 290-291.
The role of breast-feeding in child spacing seen in historical context. The effect of artificial feeding on child spacing and the impressions it creates.

——— ed. *The Medical Hazards of the Birth Control Pill.* Oak Park, Ill.: Child

and Family, 1969. 96 pp.
Uses the medical literature to document the hazards of the birth control Pill.

———— "Rhythm: I. Periodic Continence." *Child and Family* (Fall, 1968), pp. 290-295.
The lack of knowledge of or time for rhythm among doctors, and their penchant for pills rather than principles. The positive value of periodic abstinence intrinsic to the rhythm method.

———— "Rhythm: III. Population Regulation." *Child and Family* (Spring, 1969), pp. 98-101.
Population control on a worldwide basis by the rhythm method. Biases and erroneous beliefs regarding this method.

Remfry, Leonard. "The Effects of Lactation on Menstruation and Pregnation." *Transactions of the Obstetrical Society of London,* Vol. 38 (1897), pp. 22-27.

Rendu, C. *L' Eglise nous-atelle trompes?* Parish: Xavier Mappus, 1968.

Richards, Frank. *Family Planning the Natural Way.* Melbourne, Australia: Hawthorn Press, 1972. 58 pp.
An explanation of natural family planning combining mucus and temperature signs by a priest who has counseled many families.

Roetzer, Josef. "Erveiterte Basaltemperaturmessung und Empfangnisregelung." *Archiv fur Gynakologie,* 206 (1968), pp. 195-214.
This report on a combined use of basal temperature and mucus symptom finds an effectiveness at the 99 percent level (less than 1 surprise pregnancy per 100 women-years).

Schaefer, Otto. "When the Eskimo Comes to Town." *Nutrition Today* (November-December, 1971), pp. 8-16.
This physician shows how the decline in breast-feeding resulted in more than a 50 percent jump in the Eskimo birth rate and brought about more health problems for the Eskimo women and infants.

———— and J. A. Hildes. "Health of Igloolik Eskimos and Changes with Urbanization." Circumpolar Health Symposium, Oulu, Finland, June, 1971.
Shows that women aged 30-50 who raised children in camp life with prolonged breast-feeding (nursed 2-3 years) usually conceived 20 to 30 months after childbirth while the younger women exposed to urbanization and shortened lactation usually conceived 2-4 months after childbirth.

Sharman, Albert. "Ovulation After Pregnancy." *Fertility and Sterility,* Vol. II (September-October, 1951), pp. 371-393.
Ovular and anovular cycles in lactating and nonlactating women.

Slightam, Pierre E. "Remarks on Diet." *Coverline,* Vol. 2, No. 16 (Spring, 1973).
Advocates well-balanced diet as an aid to natural family planning.

Suenens, Leon Joseph Cardinal. *Love and Control.* Westminster, Md.: The Newman Press, 1967. 200 pp.
An explanation of what the Catholic Church teaches about marriage, sexuality, regulation of births, and periodic continence.

Thyma, Paul. *Fertile and Infertile Days in Married Life.* Fall River, Mass

Married Life Information Service, 1973. 63 pp.
A diagrammatic explanation of the mucus and temperature system of fertility awareness.

Tietze, Christopher. "Ranking of Contraceptive Methods by Levels of Effectiveness." Report to the American Association of Planned Parenthood Physicians, Boston, April 9-10, 1970. Published in *Advances in Planned Parenthood,* Vol. 6, pp. 117-126. Excerpta Medica International Congress Series. New York: Excerpts Medica, 1971. 180 pp.
In a descending scale of four categories of effectiveness, the associate director of the Population Council of New York ranks the postovulatory phase of the temperature method in the top group of effectiveness along with sterilization and oral contraceptives. All methods of family planning are rated.

—— and Samuel Poliakoff. "The Clinical Effectiveness of the Rhythm Method of Contraception." *Fertility and Sterility,* Vol. II (September-October, 1951), pp. 444-450.

Topkins, Paul. "The Histologic Appearance of the Endometrium During Lactation Amenorrhea and Its Relationship to Ovarian Function." *American Journal of Obstetrics and Gynecology,* Vol. VL (January-June, 1943), pp. 48-58.

Treloar, Alan E., Ruth E. Boynton, Borghild G. Behn and Byron W. Brown. "Variation of the Human Menstrual Cycle Through Reproductive Life." *International Journal of Fertility,* Vol. 12, No. 1 (January-March, 1967), Part 2, pp. 77-126.
Shows that irregularity is to be expected in any woman's menstrual history even if she is quite regular during her middle fertile years.

Udesky, Isadore. "Ovulation in Lactating Women." *Americal Journal of Obstetrics and Gynecology,* Vol. LIX (April, 1950), pp. 843-851.
Suckling in breast-feeding suppresses the ovarian cycle. Menstruation will usually appear before ovulation.

Unsworth, Richard S., et al. *Sexuality and the Human Community: A Task Force Study Document.* Philadelphia: General Assembly of the United Presbyterian Church in the U.S.A., August 1970.
A controversial study document allowing, among other things, abortion as a backstop to contraceptive failure.

Uricchio, William A., and Mary Kay Williams, eds. *Proceedings of a Research Conference on Natural Family Planning.* Washington, D.C.: The Human Life Foundation, 1973. 316 pp.
The papers and discussion presented at a conference held January 23-26, 1972, to discuss the current state of research related to natural family planning. Handy for more bibliography.

Valente, Michael F. *Sex: The Radical View of a Catholic Theologian.* New York: Bruce, 1970. 158 pp.
The author shows that his rejection of marital non-contraception logically entails the acceptance of behavior previously forbidden as contrary to the natural law,. e.g., bestiality.

van de Velde, Theodore Henry. *Uber den Zusammenhang zivischen Ovarialfunktion, Wellenbewegung und Menstrualblutung.* Haarlem, Netherlands:

F. Bohn, 1904.
A Dutch gynecologist and sexologist provides the first exact description from Europe of the changes in female body temperatures during the rhythm of the menstrual cycle.

Van Der Stappen, Guy. *Pracia de la mèthodes des temperatures.* Paris: Editions Ouvrietes, 1961. 32 pp.
A précis of the temperature method. Not personally examined.

Van Ginneken, Jeroen K. "Prolonged Breast-feeding as a Birth Spacing Method." *Studies in Family Planning,* 5:6 (June, 1974), pp. 201-206.
Reviews recent studies of lactation amenorrhea.

Vincent, Bernard. *Mèthode thermique et contraception.* Paris: Massonet Cie, 1968. 186 pp.
The temperature method of conception control considered from a medical, psychological, and sociological approach. Illustrated and diagrammed. Not personally examined.

Vincent, B., A. Aymard, M. Aymard, G. Besancon, G. Leboterf, J. Perry, and B. Vincent. *Mèthode thermique a et contraception: Approaches mèdicale et psycho-sociologique.* Paris: Masson, 1967. pp. 52-73.
Reports very high effectiveness rate for couples using a strict basal temperature system (99.99995 percent: 1 surprise pregnancy in 17,500 cycles)—quoted by C. Tietz in "ranking of Contraceptive Methods . . ."). Not personally reviewed.

———— and R. Traissac. "Continence périodique et méthode thermique." *Franc. Gynec. Obstet.,* 32:49 (1962).

Voegtli, Ottilia. *How to Use Temperature Rhythm.* Springfield, Ill.: C. C. Thomas, 1966. 69 pp.

von Hildebrand, Dietrich. *In Defense of Purity.* Chicago: Franciscan Herald Press, 1970 (originally published 1931). 142 pp.
A classic study of human love, explaining the meaning of sexuality in terms of self-donation, tenderness, affection, and reverence.

———— *The Encyclical Humanae Vitae: A Sign of Contradiction.* Chicago: Franciscan Herard Press, 1969. 89 pp.
An essay on birth control and conscience. An explanation of the nature and purpose of marriage and a reply to the objections to Humanae Vitae by the philosopher who has defended the unitive purposes of married sexuality since 1930.

———— *Man and Woman.* Logos edition. Chicago: Henry Regnery, 1966. 103 pp.
An exposition of the meaning and goodness of marital sexuality. Chapter 5 treats of birth control and distinguishes contraception from natural family planning.

Weissman, Sister M. Cosmas. "A Trial of the Ovulation Method of Family Planning in Tonga." *Lancet* (October 14, 1972), pp. 813-816. (For reader reaction, see *Lancet* [November 11, 1972], pp. 1027-1028.)
The first published report on the effectiveness of the mucus-only system of natural family planning. The report of effectiveness at the 98 percent level has been challenged.

Wessling, Frank M. "Is It Immature Loving??" *America* (May 2, 1964).
    Shows the need for a many-sided mature love in order to have a happy marriage.

Weston Laboratories, Inc. *Rhythm Can Work for You.* Ottawa, Ill.: Weston Laboratories, Inc., 1965. 6 pp.
    An explanation of various methods for determining time of ovulation, with particular emphasis on the cervical glucose test, spinnbarkeit, and physical symptoms.

W.H.O. Scientific Group. *Biology of Fertility Control by Periodic Abstinence.* W.H.O. Technical Report Series No. 360, 1967.

Zuck, R., and D. Dunean. "The Time of Ovulation in the Human Female." *American Journal of Obstetrics and Gynecology,* Vol. XXXVIII (July-December, 1939), pp. 310-315.
    Time of ovulation as determined by the measurement of the hydrogen ion concentration of vaginal secretions.